How to be Healthy, Wealthy and Wise

by
Constance Mellor
MCSP

THE C. W. DANIEL COMPANY LIMITED
60 MUSWELL ROAD, LONDON N10 2BE

First published in Great Britain
by The C.W. Daniel Company Ltd,
60 Muswell Road, London N10 2BE.

SBN 85207 138 8

Recycled Paper

The text of this book is printed on
British made recycled paper.

Set in 11pt Baskerville 2pt leaded. Printed and bound by the
White Crescent Press Ltd, Crescent Road, Luton, Beds, on
Dartex Antique Wove re-cycled paper supplied by Frank
Grunfeld Ltd, 32 Bedford Square, London WC1.

Contents

CHAPTER ONE

Prescription for Happiness

It seems to me that there is no duty we so much underrate as the duty of being happy. Only by being happy ourselves can we hope to cheer up the unhappy people – (and how many there are!) – with whom we come into contact.

Of course, without good health, happiness in the fullest sense of the word is not possible. Health is, therefore, a prerequisite of happiness.

Like most things worth having, health and happiness have to be deserved and earned. Some lucky people, through healthy parentage, are born with both; others have to learn to acquire them. In any case, both health and happiness are conditional upon three things, all of which entail a certain degree of self-denial and self-discipline. These three things are:

Right eating, right thinking, and right living.

If we eat foods that, although they may look and taste attractive, are useless as proper nourishment to the body, we suffer for it, sooner or later, irrespective of whether we commit the fault knowingly because we are slaves to our palates, or unknowingly because we are ignorant of which foods are 'health' foods and which are not. Nature does not discriminate between the people who break her laws knowingly and those who break them unknowingly; if her laws are broken, the penalty has to be paid. In the case of wrong eating, the penalty is ill-health. (See my books *Handbook of Health* and *Natural Remedies For Common Ailments*, published by C. W. Daniel.)

All life is controlled by certain inexorable laws, one of the chief of which is the law of Cause and Effect; it means that we reap what we sow. This law applies not only to our physical habits, but also to what we think and feel, inasmuch as, if we think harmful negative thoughts, or indulge in harmful negative emotions, our health is harmed by so doing.

To be happy, therefore, it is necessary to have not only a healthy body but a healthy mind and soul – body, mind, and soul being very closely related and inter-dependent. For this reason, we must try to exclude from the mind all unkind, unpleasant thoughts, and all negative harmful emotions such as worry, fear, anxiety, dread, frustration, hatred, jealousy, envy, etc, all of which adversely affect bodily health, produce stress, tension in the muscles, a disturbance of the orderly functioning of the glands, and acidity of the blood.

Healthy blood should be neutral, i.e. neither alkaline nor acid; that is why it is important to eat more of the alkaline-producing foods, (vegetables, salads, and fruits) than of the acid-producing foods (flesh-foods, starches, and sugars), because most people's blood tends to become over-acid.

Let us, therefore, learn to replace negative thoughts and emotions with positive, beneficial, and pleasant ones.

'As a man thinketh, so is he. Rise then and think with God.' Thus wrote Alexander Pope.

Much of the unhappiness in the world is due to lack of a satisfactory guide to moral behaviour – although in this respect it is perhaps only by example that one can hope to influence and guide people; words of advice about moral behaviour, unlike words of advice about nutrition and health, do not really seem to help, or to have much influence.

There are health rules, but there are no hard-and-fast rules of conduct guaranteed to bring peace of mind, success, or enjoyment of life. I can only tell you what helped *me* to find happiness; but, like the seeds in the parable of the Sower, my hints may fall on stony ground (an unreceptive mind, or a mind unready for them), and then they will bear no fruit.

Trying to explain to you how to achieve happiness is rather

like trying to teach you how to drive a car; one can only explain the mechanism of the car; it is then up to you to take the wheel of the machine into your own hands, and teach yourself to control and direct it. No one can do this *for* you.

So, here follows a brief explanation of 'the mechanism' of happiness which, I hope, will help to make clear the nature of it, and thus how to obtain it, by self-direction.

Three fundamental motives prompt *all* human behaviour. They are:
1. Egotism (which is based on self-love).
2. Malice (which is based on hate of others).
3. Compassion (which is based on love of all living creatures – human *and* animal).

Actions of moral worth can arise only from the third of these, i.e. from Compassion. *Compassion is therefore the basis of Morality.*

But, you may ask, what do you mean by Compassion? Well, I think it can best be defined as a sympathetic understanding of other people's feelings, and as the assistance we give to prevent or remove the sufferings of all living creatures, including animals. It rests upon an identification of oneself with the sufferer, so that one feels and suffers *with* him. Upon our capacity to feel and express compassion depends all our satisfaction, our well-being, our peace of mind, and our happiness.

Compassion is prompted by an inner certainty that all living creatures are One in spirit, even though they are separate entities in Time and Space. Out of the depths of one's innermost being, this certainty wells up, and it manifests itself as Compassion. Indeed, the supreme virtue, whose rule is 'Help all living creatures, as far as lies within your power', rests upon the capacity to feel Compassion. Only this virtue, free of all egoistic motives, awakens an inward happiness and contentment, gives a clear conscience, and earns the gratitude of our fellow-creatures, thus satisfying our ego's desire for appreciation.

So, two of the basic ingredients in my prescription for happiness are: an inward contentment due to a clear conscience, and the love and gratitude of one's fellow creatures.

There are, of course, other important ingredients, one of

which is pure pleasure. By this I mean the pure enjoyment derived from the sight, sound, smell, and touch of beautiful things; the pleasure we feel when we see the first snowdrop, or hear the first cuckoo in spring, or listen to wonderful music, or smell the scent of honeysuckle, or touch the velvet petals of the rose. All these things are sensual, passive pleasures; they are impractical and purposeless, divorced from any sense of duty, and unconnected with any reward, but they are essential to most people's health and happiness.

Last, but not least, of the ingredients in my prescription for happiness is an all-absorbing hobby or interest, by means of which, within the limits of one's hereditary make-up, one can express one's personality. Next to the sexual urge, the urge to express his personality is Man's strongest urge and deepest desire. He rightly feels that to express his personality is his reason for living. He should take care, however, not to attempt to accomplish things beyond his own particular capabilities, which are limited, to a great extent, by hereditary factors.

'Flying too high', and trying to accomplish things that are beyond your inborn capabilities, means that you end up frustrated, disappointed, depleted of precious nervous energy (of which we all have only the limited amount with which we were born), unhappy, and with health undermined.

Conversely, keeping within the limits of your inherent capabilities means that you end up successful, pleased, satisfied, happier, and therefore, healthier.

So, 'Do what you can; be what you are;
Shine like a glow-worm, if not like a star.' (Author unknown).

According to Aristotle, the Greek philosopher, the secret of happiness lies in doing congenial work which is of benefit to one's fellow-creatures. This is certainly part of the secret; the other part concerns one's coming to terms with the still, small voice of one's Conscience. To turn a deaf ear to this voice is to ignore God, for the voice of Conscience *is* the voice of God.

CHAPTER TWO

Stress

Stress is the wear and tear (physical and mental) that affects the body continuously from birth to death. It is the natural and inevitable result of living. All our activities (physical, mental, and emotional) involve a greater or lesser degree of stress, so we are under some degree of stress all day and every day, the amount depending upon our surroundings, our circumstances, and our individual mental and emotional make-up.

Stress is not necessarily bad for us – a little of it, like a small amount of waste-products in the blood, is a necessary stimulant, but we must be able to adapt to it successfully; if we don't, we pay the penalty of ill-health or unhappiness, or both.

To adapt successfully takes vital energy – 'adaptability energy', which we will call AE (for short). This is not the same sort of energy as the energy produced by the oxidation of food within the body. It is not produced by anything, it is inborn, and the amount you possess depends upon the amount you were born with. In other words, AE, is inherited Capital. We are all born with varying amounts, these amounts depending to a great extent upon our parentage and forebears. It is Capital that cannot be increased, but it can (and should) be used thriftily; I will explain how, later.

The causes of stress are many; here are just a few of them:
1. Strong emotions of all kinds, including intense joy, fear, anger, sorrow, frustration, worry, and all unresolved tensions, causing mental tension.

2. Physical or mental injury or shock.
3. Taking big risks of all kinds. For example, people who risk their lives, or their money, subject themselves to great stress and strain.
4. Exposure to great heat or great cold, as in the tropics or the arctic regions.
5. Heavy work (physical or mental).
6. Enforced rest or boredom. This causes more stress and strain than moderate activity.
7. An aimless life, with not enough to do or think about.
8. Unhappiness.

The body's ability to adapt to stress depends to a great extent upon its built-in, stress-fighting mechanisms, the adrenal and pituitary glands. These glands secrete 'hormones' (chemical messengers), without which the body could not stand up to the continual wear-and-tear caused by the stress of living. When these glands fail to produce sufficient hormones, 'stress' disorders may develop – disorders such as circulatory and heart diseases, digestive disorders, diseases of the kidneys, arthritis, sexual and mental derangements, etc. These are known as 'diseases of adaptation'.

Mal-adaptation to stress is also thought to be a causative factor in high blood-pressure, inflammatory conditions of the skin and the eyes, nervous diseases of many kinds, and certain types of cancer. However, some types of cancer do *not* grow well in people subjected to severe stress; in fact, the growth often undergoes considerable regression in such people, provided they are able to adapt themselves to the stress. This is because the increased secretion by their endocrine glands of anti-inflammatory hormones (ACTH and Cortisone) help to do battle against the cancer cells.

On the other hand, removal of the adrenal glands seems to retard the growth of cancer of the sex organs; this seems to suggest, therefore, that over-production of adrenal-gland hormones stimulates cancer-formation in the sex organs.

Cancers sometimes develop at the site of tissue injury, for

example, constant over-exposure to the heat-rays of the sun can cause cancer of the skin. Pipe-smoking can cause cancer of the lip, where the pipe-stem continually presses. In women, cancer of the entrance to the womb can be caused by clumsy intercourse, especially after repeated childbirth.

The relationship between stress, gland-hormones, and cancer is not clearly understood; however, it is understood sufficiently well to justify further research into the influence of stress, and of gland-hormones, upon the disease.

We should be on our guard against a shortage of essential minerals in the blood, because mineral-deficiency is tied up with the efficient working of the pituitary gland – the master-gland that controls all the other endocrine glands in the body, including the adrenal glands. For example, a magnesium deficiency means that the pituitary gland is unable to exercise proper control over the adrenal glands, and the result is an excess of adrenal-gland secretion (adrenaline) in the blood. Cortisone is one of the constituents of adrenaline and it produces a state of stress in the body – a feeling of being keyed-up and excited; an excess of it causes restlessness and sleepless nights. Natural whole-foods, such as wholewheat flour, contain sufficient magnesium for the body's normal requirements, but, to be on the safe side, it is as well to take a food-supplement containing magnesium, such as Dolomite tablets, or just a pinch of Epsom salts (Magnesium Sulphate) in your early-morning tea.

Of course, it is necessary to summon up all one's vital forces sometimes, in order to achieve something of supreme importance; however, we should not allow ourselves to get frequently carried away by over-enthusiasm, so that stress-reaction keeps us awake half the night. Gland hormones are meant to key us up for peak achievements – (in prehistoric man, for fight or flight) – they are not meant to be circulating in the blood all day and every day.

To watch our stress quota and not to exceed it is as important as to watch our alcohol quota and not exceed it; both, if exceeded, lead to intoxication – to temporary elation, followed by depression.

We can learn to keep within the limits of our stress-quota by never trying to accomplish anything beyond our powers of achievement. If we aim to achieve something that is too difficult for us, we struggle in vain, and suffer unnecessary stress due to frustration.

We must learn, therefore, to use our capital – our adaptability energy – wisely and carefully, because we have only a limited amount of it. In planning your life – *and* your day – remember that variety should be the keynote, for not only is variety 'the spice of life'; it is a prolonger of life, and it is an equaliser – it equalises stress, ensuring equal wear-and-tear on all parts of the body and of the mind. Over-use of any one part of you means that that part wears out sooner than the other parts.

In an ability to adapt successfully to the constantly-changing conditions, and to the stresses and strains of everyday life, lies the secret of Health, Happiness and of Longevity.

Ageing – the wearing-out of the body – is due largely to the stresses of life which gradually exhaust our adaptability energy. However, by learning to use our AE wisely, and by eating sparingly of natural rather than refined foods, we can prolong our life-span, avoid ill-health in old age, and die peacefully, of natural causes.

(For further reading about stress, see *The Stress of Life* by Dr Hans Selye, MD, published by Longmans.)

CHAPTER THREE

Conservation of Energy

Economy of effort – that is the keynote of the teachings of Dr Matthias Alexander, who, in the late 1920s, started a school for children at his country home in Kent. He taught them how to make all the simple everyday movements such as sitting-down, getting-up, standing, walking, etc, with the minimum expenditure of effort, thus conserving vital energy.

All movements, he said, should be under the conscious control of the mind. He believed that, in order to keep healthy and vital, we should all conserve energy in every possible way, and that one big way in which we *can* do this is by what he called 'the right use of self'. He believed that the conscious mind has the power to control and to regenerate body-function. (See *Inside Yourself* by Louise Morgan, published by Hutchinson, which gives a very lucid explanation of his teachings.)

Most people (including children) put far too much effort into nearly every movement they make, thus wasting precious energy and becoming tired, so that they find themselves unable to 'pay attention' in class. Conscious control of one's movements, coupled with erectness of one's head, alters all that. This erectness of one's head, (the back of which should be in a continuous straight line with the spinal column, neither poked forward nor pushed back) frees the complex of muscles at the back of the neck where the neck joins the head, which is the centre of 'the primary control'. This control-centre co-ordinates all body movements. It is well-developed in animals because they use it so much, but in Man it has fallen into disuse, and is, therefore, weak. It can, however, be strengthened by use. In order to use it properly, it must be freed of the pressure of the muscle-complex in which it resides, by keeping the back of the head erect, in a straight line with the spinal column. This means that the chin should be slightly drawn in, but the head should not feel 'held' in this position; it should simply feel poised on the top of the spine, of which it is a continuation.

There is, as Dr Alexander points out, a very marked contrast between the unhappy condition of present-day civilised man and the happy condition of animals, who are obviously happy just to be alive; who perform, with ease and grace and the minimum amount of energy-expenditure, complicated movements which call for perfect co-operation of body and mind. Think of the squirrel, how he leaps from branch to branch of a tree, and from one tree to another. There are, of course, human acrobats who can do similar things, but they are few and far between.

Present-day man has failed to keep pace with his rapidly-changing environment which is the result of scientific progress, and he is maladjusted mentally to the changed (and changing) world around him. His life is often dominated by fear of one sort or another – fear of modern inventions, fear of war and of the atom bomb, fear of food-shortage, etc, and it is fear that undermines success, saps self-confidence, and causes failure – in the mental as well as the physical sphere.

Many people suffer from a fear-complex. With some people it is fear of silence (they must have background music or noise of some sort around them); with others it is fear of solitude, or fear of the dark, or of confined spaces, or of illness, or of the future, or of death. Whatever the particular fear, (or fears) it causes tension of mind and body, and a consequent lack of co-ordination of the two, and this (as well as fear) leads to failure. Failure leads to frustration, which leads to unhappiness, which leads to symptoms of ill-health (such as insomnia, or constipation, or fatigue, or restlessness and nerviness), and ill-health leads to the taking of medicinal drugs or of strong drink – perhaps even to crime, or insanity, or suicide.

Despite surface improvements in the nation's health, a high proportion of present-day ill-health is therefore functional, arising as the direct result of a fear-complex and of the wrong use of self, and it can be put right by the right use of self, as taught by Dr Alexander. This right use of self frees the body of tension, and so, to a great extent, of fear.

The Director of an Institute of Medical Research in Melbourne has said that disease should not be tackled by new drugs and new remedies, but by the study of how intrinsic factors (i.e. self-caused factors) influence its onset.

What we really need, therefore, is not more hospitals, more nurses, and more drugs, but more trained people (doctors and medical auxiliaries) to teach people (especially children) the right use of their bodies, together with other natural methods of 'disease prevention' such as correct nutrition. The need for 'disease treatment' would then diminish, half our hospitals and mental institutions would be able to close down, and all (or nearly all) medicines (except natural ones, like herbs and biochemic minerals) could be thrown into the sea (but Heaven help the fishes!).

The training for such 'disease-prevention' teaching should be part of the curriculum in medical training schools, so that all doctors could teach their patients not only the right use of self, as first taught with such outstanding success in functional diseases by Dr Alexander, but also the right way to feed.

As things are at present, such training is still not included in the medical curricula (doctors are trained to be simply disease-treaters, not disease-preventers), despite the fact that, as long ago as 1937, it was suggested to the authority responsible for the selection of subjects to be studied by medical students that such training should be included. It was strongly urged in a letter published in the *British Medical Journal* which was signed by nineteen eminent London consultants (including the then Vice-president of the BMA) but nothing came of their urgent suggestion, and, to this day, no training is given in medical training schools either in the subject of nutrition or in the Alexander technique, a knowledge of which would enable doctors to prevent (and cure) many functional *and* organic diseases. The drug industry donates huge grants to medical training schools where the use by the students of its new 'wonder' drugs is encouraged.

Herbal medicine is no longer popular – it is not as money-making as medicinal drugs; also its effects are longer-lasting and more curative; it is therefore less lucrative. How true the old saying: 'Love of money is the root of all evil'.

CHAPTER FOUR

All Work and No Play

There is a very close connection between disease and the prevailing social system.

Civilisation restricts Man's natural instincts, especially his sexual instinct. The result is that his personality – his Psyche, as it is sometimes called – is denied sufficient opportunity for relaxation and repose, and this inevitably leads to a state of mental tension, of anxiety, indefinable dread (though dread of what, he does not know), and restlessness.

Just as his physical body needs regular periods of rest, so also does his Psyche. He needs to divest himself of it sometimes – to lose himself in something or someone. This satisfies a natural desire of the Psyche to relax. Such instinctive and natural desire can be satisfied by sexual union with a loved one; it can also be satisfied by the contemplation of beauty in Nature and the Arts; by pleasure in general; and by sleep, though self-assertive people find difficulty in surrendering themselves to sleep, in overcoming the initial phase of physical relaxation, in order to reach the deep phase in which they can surrender their personalities completely.

Civilisation lays too much stress on the pursuit of long-term aims, difficult to attain – such things as attainment of wealth, power, fame, and success in one's profession or social sphere – and too little stress on the importance of satisfying simpler, more immediate and fundamental desires and instincts, particularly the creative instinct.

Craftsmen and their creations are no longer needed. It is an age of machines – of impersonal industry and mass-production; so Man has to divert his natural creative instincts into other channels, making them the motive-power behind long-term distant aims, the fulfilment of which is sometimes deferred for years. This is all highly unnatural and frustrating, because long-deferred fulfilment of aims means long-deferred satisfaction for the Psyche. The consequence of this is, quite often, physical ill-health.

Some of Man's goals should therefore be easily-attained ones, bringing pleasure, and consequent rest to the Psyche.

Sensual pleasures are – or should be – part of a balanced life. Among sensual pleasures I include the pleasure of acquiring skill in games and sports; the pleasure of music-making and other arts; the pleasure of creating things with one's brain or one's hands (or both); the pleasures of sight, smell, and touch; the pleasures of sexual love; and the pleasure of giving oneself up to sleep. In all these ways a very necessary let-up and rest for the Psyche is provided, which, like the body, must have its off-duty times. Such pleasurable relaxation is the key that unlocks the door to harmony of mind and body – and thus to health, health being an attribute of a harmonious Psyche.

Pleasure is a powerful therapeutic agent; it contributes to good health, and helps to heal. An illustration of this is the fact that we put flowers in a sick-room because we know that the sight and smell of beautiful things gives sensual pleasure to the invalid, and that this sensual pleasure satisfies and rests his (or her) Psyche.

Beautiful music in beautiful surroundings has the same effect. It is used nowadays in mental hospitals, just as it was in Greece, in times BC – Greek physicians made a study of their patients' personalities, because they believed, as enlightened present-day doctors are coming to believe, that many of Man's illnesses and diseases are caused to a great extent by a lack of harmony between the instinctive and the reasoning parts of his brain – between his autonomic nervous-system and his central nervous-system.

Great things are achieved and great problems are solved not necessarily by people who make great efforts of will. Usually, people whose autonomic and central nervous systems work together in complete harmony and are perfectly synchronised, achieve most. The lack of tension between the instinctive and the reasoning parts of their brain enables them to concentrate on the job in hand; they achieve an even and balanced functioning of mind and body, and a harmonising of their personality with the world around them.

It usually comes about, therefore, that great things are achieved by simple people, people who take simple pleasure in everyday things which provide them with outlets for their natural impulses. They are thereby enabled to maintain a nice state of balance between their autonomic nervous system and their central nervous system, which results in a relaxed calmness of mind, and a healthy body. They instinctively know that 'All work and no play makes Jack a dull – and a sick – boy'.

CHAPTER FIVE

Powerful Possessions

'Self-reverence, Self-knowledge, Self-control,
These three alone lead life to sovereign power.'

(Tennyson)

An equally important possession, in my opinion, is *Self-help*, because, as we all know, 'God helps them who help themselves'. This applies particularly in illness, when perhaps you are fighting for your life. The battle is as good as won if you have a firm belief in your body's recuperative powers, all physical treatment (diet, medicines, etc) being of secondary importance to 'the will to live' – indeed, many of the medicinal drugs prescribed nowadays by most orthodox doctors will hinder rather than help the body's self-healing efforts. Drugs treat symptoms rather than causes, and give more work for the eliminative organs to do, when these organs are already working overtime.

On the other hand, the *right* kind of medicines – herbal, bio-chemic, homoeopathic, etc – combined with correct feeding (or with fasting, followed by correct feeding) can help the body's self-healing efforts. Also, great help comes from the positive vibrations generated by a positive mind and will. These vibrations create positive electro-magnetic currents in the body, and these stimulate and incite the millions of tiny cells, doing battle in the inflamed and sick part of the body, to fight harder.

The victory in disease is therefore conditional not only upon correct feeding of the body and upon natural remedies, but upon complete faith in the body's ability to cure itself – as, of course, it can, and usually does.

Self-knowledge

This is usually thought of as knowledge of how the mind works, but a knowledge of how the body works and of its needs is of more importance really. Such knowledge enables us to keep healthy, and the chances are that if our bodies are healthy, our minds and our emotions will be healthy too, the relationship between body and mind being a very close one.

> *'Know then thyself; presume not God to scan.*
> *The proper study of Mankind is Man.'*

Our education authorities should be reminded of these words, (which were written by Alexander Pope in his *Essay on Man*) and should be pressed to include the teaching of elementary physiology and anatomy to teenagers of both sexes. Correct feeding, the value of fresh air and exercise, and the art of relaxed movement (as taught by Dr Alexander), should also be taught in all schools. Books on 'health' subjects, such as nutrition, should be available in school lending-libraries, and 'health' lectures should include advice about Nature-cure 'health' books for home-reading. It seems to me that the teaching of sex knowledge, other than a knowledge of the sex organs and of how they function, (which would be included in the physiology lectures) is neither necessary nor advisable.

Owing to an absence of 'health' education, there is much suffering in the world, as well as much unnecessary spending of public money. The National Health Service spends millions of pounds a year on medicinal drugs alone, the demand for which, I am convinced, would gradually decrease as health education increased.

Where a knowledge of the mind is concerned, it should be realised that the mind consists of a conscious and an unconscious part. The conscious mind makes decisions and deals with all the problems, worries, etc, of everyday life, although more often than is realised it is prompted and helped by the unconscious mind, which is a storehouse of memories, and the residence of the soul, from whence emerges 'the still small voice of conscience'.

It sometimes happens that the conscious mind, after trying very hard to battle with some insoluble problem or to resolve some worry, feels it cannot go on trying any longer – that it is all too difficult. If and when this happens, it should hand everything over to the unconscious mind, which will deal with it very efficiently if given a little time and not hurried. Give your conscious mind a complete rest from whatever it is that is worrying you – don't *try* to cope with it consciously if you have already honestly tried hard and failed. Then one morning, when you wake, the solution of your problem will be clear to you, clear as daylight; your unconscious mind has dealt with it, found the solution, and pushed this through the letter-box of your conscious mind.

An aid to Self-knowledge is an understanding of the doctrines and teachings of Theosophy. These are explained very clearly and simply by Harry Benjamin in *Everybody's Guide to Theosophy*, published by Health for All Publishing Company.

Self-control

This can be defined as an ability to stop short of excess and exhaustion. If we carry anything beyond exhaustion-point, we suffer from enervation, which is another word for loss of vital energy (vitality). It is enervation that is the real underlying cause of *all* ill-health and disease, because it saps the body's powers of resistance, and undermines the body's defence mechanisms against microbial attack.

Also when the body is enervated, it is unable, through lack of vitality, to eliminate toxic substances (the self-made sort, *and* the sort that are ingested with the foods eaten and the air breathed), and these, circulating in the bloodstream, start to ferment, causing a fever in the blood. This the body tries to throw off through one (or more) of its mucous membranes, the membrane chosen being the one that is most irritated by the poison-gas produced by the fermentation of the toxins. The common cold is an example of an irritation of the nasal mucous membrane, which is caused primarily by a toxic state of the blood, the 'cold' germ being only the secondary cause of the trouble, for the simple reason that no germ or virus can live and multiply in a clean bloodstream; it can (and does) live and multiply *only* in an unclean one.

Thus, an unclean bloodstream, which is the result of inefficient elimination of toxic materials from the system, is the underlying cause of all infections.

In normal health, purging of the system, *by* the system, of accumulated waste products and toxins takes place quite easily and naturally through the organs of elimination (the bowels, kidneys, skin, and lungs). It is only when these organs are clogged or over-worked, or when the body is enervated and lacks vitality, that elimination becomes inefficient, thereby lowering the body's resistance to infections and disease.

Let us remember, therefore, that any 'activity' which we continue to the point of exhaustion saps vital energy, causing Enervation (loss of vitality) and consequent retention of toxins in the system, and that this retention of toxins is the cause not only of minor ailments such as colds, but that it paves the way to more serious illnesses, and even, eventually, to disease. (The word 'activity' is here used in its widest sense to cover all kinds of mental and emotional activities, as well as physical ones such as eating and drinking.)

The need for hospitals (other than hospitals for accidents, deformities, and emergency surgery) would decrease rapidly if Man learned self-control. As it is, he is a slave to his appetites; he lives to eat, rather than eats to live, much disease being caused by over-indulgence in food and drink.

Likewise it is certain that the divorce courts would soon close down if love between married couples were not killed, (as it so often is) by over-indulgence in sexual pleasures.

CHAPTER SIX

National Health – (or Sub-Health?)

In view of the fact that orthodox methods of healing do not seem able to cope with the increase in diseases of all kinds (especially degenerative diseases), and that it is the duty of the medical profession to heal, the time has come, surely, when unorthodox methods should be given a trial.

The whole conventional armoury of medical weapons should be inspected and examined, and some of the obsolete ones (like vaccination and other forms of immunisation) scrapped, and replaced by newly-forged ones like biochemistry, chiropractic, osteopathy, radionics, etc, supplemented by naturopathy, which is basic to all other therapies, and homoeopathy. (All these therapies are described in detail in *Fringe Medicine* by Brian Inglis, published by Faber and Faber; and in *The Frontiers of Healing* by Geoffrey Murray, published by Max Parrish.)

We need medical therapy that is compatible with natural laws; what we have is drugs. These just suppress the symptoms without doing anything towards removing the cause of the symptoms. All the unorthodox therapies mentioned above (with the exception of homoeopathy) are excluded from the National Health Service. They should, of course, be included, so that people who wish to be treated by naturopathy, or osteopathy, or one of the other unorthodox methods, *can* be, without having to pay private fees for treatment.

First and foremost, though, we need laws to ensure the purity of our foods, of our drinking water, and of the air we breathe, which means that we need dedicated men and women to enforce these laws. Without such laws, and without a big drive at international level to improve the soil in which our foods are grown, all medical treatments (orthodox *and* unorthodox) are a futile waste of time and of the nation's money. They are comparable to bailing out the water from a leaking boat without first stopping the leak. Mineral-rich, naturally-fertilised soil, and whole uncontaminated foods, water, and air, are the basic and essential pre-conditions for good health; without them, there can only be sub-health – as there is at present.

If the soil in which our foods are grown is sick and exhausted (and, as the result of bad husbandry and of greedy growing-for-profit, most soil in Great Britain, and elsewhere, is), it can produce only sick crops and sick animals, deficient in essential minerals, trace-elements, etc. This means that the people who eat these deficiency foods will also be far from fit and well, because their food is not supplying them with the vital substances they need for good health. (See Chapter 15 of my book *Handbook of Health* – also *The Soil and Health* by Sir Albert Howard, *The Living Soil* by Lady Eve Balfour, and *The Earth's Green Carpet* by Lady Howard.)

From birth to death, the majority of present-day people never experience the taste of natural, whole, uncontaminated foods – foods that have not been tampered with in one way or another. Whole natural foods are in short supply and difficult to come by, except at health foods shops (and the number of these is all too few), so it is not altogether their own fault that people are slowly poisoning themselves, day by day, with the foods they eat (not to mention the water they drink, which is doctored with all sorts of chemicals nowadays).

But, of course, most people do not give much thought to what they put inside themselves, or take much trouble to obtain whole natural foods; they take the line of least resistance and buy their foods from local shops. Usually these foods (unless they come from a health-food shop) are not 'health' foods, indeed, they may well be not only 'deficiency' foods but contaminated foods, because nowadays meat, poultry, vegetables, and fruit have generally been chemically treated, and they therefore contain chemical residues, many of which are poisonous.

Present-day food is flavourless too – it lacks 'real' flavour because it has been fed on 'artificials'. Commercially-grown vegetables and fruits, broiler chickens, veal, and battery eggs, all these are particularly tasteless, partly because they are artificially fed, and partly because the conditions under which they are produced and reared are highly unnatural – *and* (in the case of the animals) cruel. (The unnatural and cruel methods used in factory-farming have been revealed by Mrs Harrison in her book *Animal Machines*, published by Vincent Stuart Ltd.)

Health begins in the soil. It is not surprising, therefore, that ill-health and disease of all kinds is on the increase, not only in humans but in animals and plants too. In the case of humans, this increase could be partly due to 'soul-sickness', of which there is abundant evidence everywhere, but by far the greater part of it is due to 'soil-sickness', to unnatural and deficiency foods, and to the poor-quality fodder given to food-producing animals, such as cows and hens. Even people of strong healthy parentage seem to enjoy only sub-health, whilst others, less fortunate genetically, seem to be permanently far from fit and well, and are frequently in hospital, or having medical treatment at home.

By providing hospitals for the care and treatment of the sick, the Government pursues a policy of 'cure'. But prevention is better than cure, as everyone knows; indeed, it is the *only* cure for some illnesses. The Government should therefore make itself responsible for the prevention, as well as for the cure, of disease. This would mean devoting some of the millions of pounds it spends annually on disease-treatment to treatment of the soil in which our foods are grown. It would mean giving more financial help to the Ministry of Agriculture for country-wide compost-making and sewage-utilisation schemes. Such schemes would not only avoid sewage-pollution of our rivers, from which much of our drinking-water comes, but would encourage growers of food-crops to use compost and sewage-sludge instead of artificial fertilisers which, by themselves, do *not* give the plant all that it needs. If 'artificials' are used without organic fertilisers such as manure, compost, sewage-sludge, etc, the nice chemical balance of the soil is upset, and the valuable soil-population – the unpaid workers (the beneficial bacteria) who fertilise the soil – are largely destroyed.

A Government 'prevention' policy should also include financial help for research into biological methods of plant-pest control. These would replace the need for poison-sprays which are widely used on nearly all food-crops nowadays. These poison-sprays destroy many useful forms of wild life including bees, birds, and other natural predators. Their poisonous residues are absorbed by the crops onto which they are sprayed, and ingested therefore by the animals and the people who eat the crops. Crops are attacked by pests and disease only when their resistance to disease has been weakened by deficiency feeding. (This is true also of animals *and* of human beings.)

Many eminent soil-scientists, including Sir Robert McCarrison, F. Newman Turner, Jorian Jenks, and Professor Schuphan, have demonstrated the superiority of farming methods that use natural organic manures and compost to feed the soil, rather than artificial fertilisers, by being able to dispense with all poisonous sprays on their crops – the crops being so healthy that pests and diseases did not attack them. Their successful methods of cultivation are well known to the Ministry of Agriculture, but the Ministry shows no signs of any intention to adopt them. Powerful arguments against their adoption are, no doubt, brought to bear on the Ministry by the chemical industries who manufacture the sprays; they know that if 'organic' methods of agriculture *were* widely adopted, chemical sprays, etc, would no longer be needed, neither would artificial fertilisers – and this would cripple the industry.

Other 'prevention' measures that should be taken by the Government are concerned with the water we drink, and the air we breathe. Our rivers, from which much of our water comes, are polluted by sewage, also by effluents from domestic and industrial premises; these effluents contain detergents which it is well-nigh impossible to wholly eradicate from the water. The Government should make it illegal to use rivers for the disposal of sewage (and other wastes) and should start a national sewage-utilisation scheme to replace sewage-disposal.

The air we breathe is polluted not only by fall-out from atom-bomb testing, but by poisonous fumes from factory and domestic chimneys, and from motor and aeroplane exhausts. The Government cannot, of course, be expected to control atomic scientists (only a change of heart in Man will banish the atom bomb), but it could and should control all the other sources of pollution, especially exhaust-fumes from motors, because it is believed by many eminent cancer specialists that these are a more significant cause of lung cancer than is smoking. Sir Walter Fergusson-Hannay, an eminent cancer specialist, was a non-smoker, yet he died of cancer of the lungs, which he believed was largely due to inhalation of poisonous fumes in the atmosphere of city streets. I think what we all want to know is why the Government does not make filters on car exhaust-pipes compulsory.

If the Government put into operation the above 'prevention' measures, the need for hospitals, other than hospitals for accidents, deformities, and the mentally sick, would gradually disappear. In fact, if people ate only non-flesh, uncontaminated, 'whole' foods (in their natural raw state as far as possible), and drank natural spring-water or distilled water, it is more than likely that degenerative diseases, including cancer, would decrease rapidly, and would soon become merely a matter of medical history.

CHAPTER SEVEN

Eating for Health

We eat to live, but as a wise man once said, 'It is not the food in our life that matters; what matters is the life in our food'. Whole, unrefined, uncooked foods contain the germ of life, without which food is useless for nourishing the millions of cells of which the body is composed; indeed, any other sort of food, being dead, is worse than useless – it simply gives the digestive organs work to do without providing the necessary energy with which to do it. Fragmented foods, i.e. foods that have been split up and have had some of their vital parts removed (such as whole-wheat that has had its bran and its germ removed; sugar-cane that has been bleached to make it white and therefore de-mineralised), also foods that have been subjected to heat treatment or 'processed' – these are 'deficiency' foods that any wise housewife or catering officer, with an inborn sense of the True and the Good, will instinctively reject. They are the foodless foods which are not only deprived of their precious and vital parts, but subjected to 'processing', to sterilisation, and to chemicalisation, in order to preserve them for a longer time, i.e. to give them a longer shelf-life.

The manufacturers of these 'dead' products – the 'vested interests' that finance their production, whose only concern is to make fat profits, and who couldn't care less about people's health (or lack of health) – these are the real culprits; it is they who are responsible for the present-day widespread ill-health in the world. Our health has been taken out of our own hands and out of the hands of our doctors, and is largely in their hands.

Unfortunately, ill-health cannot be cured by medical drugs, for the simple reason that these do not make-good the nutritional deficiencies that cause it. Indeed, to a very great extent, medical drugs actually *contribute* to ill-health and disease, by allowing the real cause, deficiency foods (and these include cooked foods) to be overlooked.

Deficiency feeding gives warning signs and symptoms, such as stomach and bowel disorders, migraine, tiredness, nerviness, an inability to cope and to feel alive and well, etc. These signs and symptoms are suppressed if medical drugs are taken, so that their real cause is not suspected and not treated, and gradually the sufferer's health gets worse, and eventually (after many years perhaps) disease becomes established in his (or her) body.

It is not generally realised that the body can be over-fed yet under-nourished, and that imperfectly nourished body-cells deteriorate and become diseased. Foods that are lacking in inorganic minerals and 'trace-elements' (the minerals that our vegetables, our cereals, our fruits and nuts and seeds contain – or *should* contain if the soil in which they are grown contains them) are useless as body-building material, just as building stones are useless without a stone-mason to build them into a structure; in other words, the organic content of our food is useless as nourishment without the inorganic minerals. This brings us to a realisation of the importance of soil fertility, and of the truth of the saying 'Health begins in the soil'. A deficiency soil, due to bad husbandry and/or an ignorance of soil science, can produce only 'deficiency' crops lacking in one or more of the essential minerals or 'trace-elements', and 'deficiency' crops are 'deficiency' foods. These will be turned into *doubly* deficient food when (as already explained) they have been tampered with (i.e. fragmented, processed, and chemicalised) by food manufacturers. There is, therefore, a need for growing our own vegetables, salads, herbs, fruits, nuts and seeds, using home-made compost and other natural fertilisers such as pulverised seaweed, bone-meal, etc, on the soil in which they are grown.

Commercially-grown vegetables and fruits are generally deficient in essential minerals and trace-elements because the soil in which they are grown is deficient in these things. Mother Earth, like any human mother carrying a child (or children), must be fed properly if she is to produce healthy offspring, and commercial growers do not usually feed their soils properly; they use mostly chemical fertilisers, and these upset the nice chemical balance of the soil, and destroy earthworms and other valuable soil creatures that help to fertilise the soil.

There is a need, too, for eating more raw and fewer cooked foods. Man is the only animal who cooks his food before eating it, thereby rendering it unsuitable for assimilation and for nourishment of the body, because cooking destroys the vitamins and digestive enzymes in the food. This applies particularly to protein foods (meat, cheese, eggs and milk) all of which are rendered not only indigestible and devalued by cooking but also positively harmful.* So, any protein foods that cannot be eaten raw should be omitted from the diet. This means that meat (and other flesh foods) will have to be omitted because they are unpalatable and revolting if uncooked.

Fortunately, some of us realise that we don't *have* to eat dead animals and lifeless, fragmented, processed, chemicalised foods that have been killed stone-dead in abattoirs, factories, and laboratories – that whole, unspoilt substitutes for meat *are* available for the seeking, mostly at health-food shops and the health-food department of large stores such as Harrods of London, and Selfridges. In most big towns there is nowadays a health-food shop, where foods containing the vital nutrients required by the human body are obtainable. And not only foods; food-supplements are also obtainable at these shops. These make-good any mineral or vitamin deficiency there might be in the foods, a deficiency probably due to a deficiency in the soil in which the food was grown. It is, therefore, advisable to shop at a health-food shop where natural unrefined foods and food-supplements are obtainable.

*The albumen in flesh foods is decomposed, by cooking, into toxic compounds.

Flesh foods contain all the essential amino-acids needed by the body; for this reason, they are spoken of as 'complete' proteins. Most of the substitutes for flesh foods (such things as nuts, seeds, cereals, pulses, etc) lack one (or more) of the essential amino-acids and are, therefore, not 'complete' proteins. Of the non-flesh foods, only milk, cheese, eggs, dried milk and brewers' yeast are 'complete' protein-foods. Yet 'complete' protein is absolutely essential to the maintenance of good health. The great problem is, therefore, how to be healthy on a vegetarian diet. The answer to this can be found by reading my book *Natural Remedies for Common Ailments* (pages 214–24). On page 222 there is a table showing the comparative values of all the various vegetarian foods (in terms of their protein content) and, by studying this, the reader will see how to combine 'incomplete' proteins in such a way as to obtain a 'complete' one. This is based upon the fact that the essential amino-acid lacking in one of them will be found to be present in another, and that, if these two are combined and eaten together, they will then form a 'complete' protein-food.

CHAPTER EIGHT

Back to the Land

A garden is a lovesome thing, God wot;
Rose-plot, fringed pool, ferned grot –
The veriest school of Wisdom.
And yet the fool contends that God is not.
Not God, in gardens when the eve is cool?
Nay, but I have a sign;
'Tis very sure God walks in mine.

What inspired words, written by the nineteenth-century poet T. E. Brown! And, of course, a garden is not only a lovesome thing, it is a most important aid to good health and contentment of mind, in that it provides us with out-door exercise, bringing us into close contact with Nature and all the natural forces of sun, wind, water, and earth. It also provides us with vegetables, fruits, nuts, seeds, and herbs, all of which are rich in all the vitamins and minerals our bodies need and *must* have if they are to remain healthy.

But our soil can feed properly the crops we grow in it only if we feed *it* properly; it can't go on, year after year, producing mineral-rich crops if the minerals which the crops take from it are not replaced. They are best replaced by compost (weeds and vegetable waste-materials, mixed together to form a heap, which rots down to a sweet-smelling substance, full of all the things essential to plant-life). This kind of plant-food is vastly superior to artificial fertilisers out of a bag.

Hippocrates, doctor of medicine about 2,500 years ago, in ancient Greece, is known to have said 'Let food be your medicine'. Nowadays this advice (which is often quoted by present-day doctors) is quite useless advice, for the simple reason that, unless you grow it yourself, present-day food lacks many vitally important minerals, trace-elements, and vitamins. It is useless, therefore, to prescribe, say, carrot-juice, in the belief that it will cure some ailment (such as gastric ulcer), unless you know that the carrots used for the making of the juice were grown on mineral-rich, composted soil. It stands to reason that our crops are only as rich in mineral nutrients as is the soil in which they are grown – that they cannot extract nutrients from a soil that is deficient in them.

So, grow your own crops, as far as possible, in naturally-fertilised soil; then you have a medicine chest, full of the most valuable medicaments, at your back-door. These are of far greater value to you than any medicine your NHS doctor can prescribe.

Wheat, of course, we cannot grow in our back-garden, but we can get good wholewheat flour, (made from wholewheat grains, grown on composted soil), at all health-food shops, and with this we can (and should) make our own bread and cakes.

What a pity it is that only about 25 per cent of the population are occupied in agriculture and horticulture and that the remaining 75 per cent, who are engaged in industry and commerce, have to live unnatural sedentary lives, in towns and cities, in fume-laden air. Until about 200 years ago, it was just the reverse – 75 per cent of the people lived and worked on the land and were far healthier and happier in consequence. The invention of machinery is largely responsible for the flow of people from country to town.

It is thought by some eminent historians that the decline and fall of the great nations in the history of the world has been due, fundamentally, to neglect of the soil and its proper cultivation – i.e. to bad husbandry. This was thought to be the real cause of the fall of the great Roman Empire, and it will probably be the cause of the fall of the British Empire. For empires cannot be built and maintained by improperly-nourished people. Brains as well as 'brawn' are needed for the efficient running of an empire, and the human brain cannot function efficiently and clearly if it is nourished with blood which is lacking in vitally important minerals, trace-elements, etc.

It is the gradual deterioration in the physical, mental, and moral health of a nation that is the fundamental cause of that nation's decline. But our health is basically dependent upon the proper cultivation of the soil in which our foods are grown, so we cannot expect to be an A.1 nation if we have to eat foods grown in an impoverished C.3 soil.

The Government pursues a short-sighted policy in spending vast sums on money on the *treatment* of disease, and comparatively little on its *prevention*. Much more should be spent on research into the causes of disease, in order to put into operation a nation-wide 'prevention of disease' programme.

It should be widely realised that prevention is the only sure cure, and, with this in mind, people should be encouraged to cultivate their own small plot of garden and grow their own crops – or, if they haven't got a garden, to rent an allotment.

Gardening – especially the growing of food-crops, nuts, and fruits – has been Man's natural occupation since pre-historic times, and should continue to be at least his part-time hobby. Allotments within easy reach of their town should be available to town-dwellers with no gardens (land should be set aside by the Government for this purpose).

Our present social system, based, as it is, upon machines, upon the great masses of workers (the proletariat), and upon the exploitation of these two factors, is an entirely unnatural one.

So long as Man lives in an unnatural artificial environment where there is a deficiency of fresh air, sun, natural foods, and no quiet or freedom, and so long as there exists the exploitation of Man by Man, there will never be social peace and security, and we shall always have diseases and epidemics, revolutions, and wars. For present society is out of harmony with natural laws. This fact implies the existence of two antagonistic forces – the force of Nature, and the force of present Society. The force of Nature is the stronger, and will, of course, win in the end. The whole of humanity is only a small superstructure living on the surface of our planet, which, with the rest of the solar system, obeys natural laws, and these natural laws, in the course of endless evolution, always destroy everything that is out of harmony with them.

Similarly, no individual can have good health and long life if he lives contrary to natural laws; nor can any social system exist for long if it is out of harmony with these laws – it is destroyed, just as the individual is destroyed.

There would be a natural human society if 75 per cent of the people occupied themselves with cultivation of the land and 25 per cent with industry and commerce. But we see 75 per cent of the population concentrated in cities, following various unhealthy occupations, and this concentration is largely responsible for the biological degeneration of the human race. Even the 25 per cent who *do* cultivate the land use wrong methods of husbandry, producing cereals to feed animals, which are then killed to feed humans.

If, instead of breeding animals and raising crops to feed them, our farmers were to raise fruit and nuts and cereals to feed direct to humans, they could earn five times as much money for one quarter the work. And the improvement in the nation's health would be enormous. But, because meat is mistakenly thought to be an essential part of Man's diet, the best part of our land is used as grazing-land for animals destined for slaughter. It could feed millions more people if it were used for growing cereals and crops for 'direct' feeding of the population.

Man has strayed far from his natural path! He will have to get back to it, or become extinct.

CHAPTER NINE

Crimes Against Creation

The vast majority of people lack what seems to me to be one of the most important human virtues – namely, compassion – without which all their other good qualities are, in my opinion, comparatively worthless.

Compassion is the basis of morality. People who doubt this should read *The Basis of Morality* by the great philosopher Schopenhauer. It will convince them. So, too, will Esme Wynne-Tyson's book *The Philosophy of Compassion*.

The vast majority of people with whom one comes into contact appear to be completely unconcerned about everyone and everything that is outside the circle of their own small world. Within this small world, their main concern seems to be the satisfying of their palates, of their sexual desires, and of their creature-comforts, plus the pursuit of diversions and amusements for the mind, in the form of television, films, theatres, card-games, and novel-reading. As long as their food and drink is forthcoming, they do not give a thought to where it comes from or how it is obtained; to the diabolical cruelty that is involved in the slaughter of animals for food, and to the degradation of the men who do the killing. The same can be said about their creature-comforts, such as coal fires, fur coats, etc, and about their beautifiers (cosmetics, perfumes, soaps, lotions, etc).

The price paid in animal suffering for all of these things is a very high one, but this does not concern most people; it's only the price they pay for them in the shops that concerns them. You may say 'But most people are not aware of the price paid in animal suffering'; to which the obvious reply is 'If *I* am aware of it, *they* could, and should, be'.

Where coal is concerned, human as well as animal suffering is involved. A miner's life is an unnatural one, his health suffers in consequence, and he usually dies at an early age. So, too, do the little pit-ponies which, like the miners, spend the best part of their lives in the bowels of the earth, are worked to death, and die of exhaustion.

As for the trapping and killing of wild animals for their beautiful skins, and of whales for their fats to make soaps, cosmetic oils, margarine, etc, this is nothing short of barbarous. Baby seals are clubbed on the head, but this only stuns them, and they are then skinned alive, in full view of their helpless, demented mothers. The *Daily Mirror* on 15th April, 1967, devoted a full front page to an illustrated article on the diabolical cruelties of the sealing industry. Other informative articles and leaflets can be obtained from The Animal Defence League, 52 Dean Street, London W1.

Whales are killed by electric harpoons which are thrown at them from whaling gun boats, but, as these weapons do not kill instantaneously, the poor creatures lash about in agony, sometimes for many hours, before they finally die in extreme agony.

Civet cats are tortured, to produce a flow of their sex-gland secretion. This is used in the manufacture of expensive perfumes. The wealthy people who buy such perfumes are probably unaware of this; such practices are kept very secret, and the majority of people do not know about them.

Geese are forcibly fed with corn to make their livers swell, so that, when they are killed, a bigger weight of *pâté-de-fois-gras* (which is made from goose-livers) can be produced.

Vivisection (experiments on animals) is another very cruel form of animal-exploitation practised in the name of Science by chemists, scientists, and research workers. Many of the experiments are very cruel, involving surgery (sometimes without anaesthetics) and the implantation of diseased tissue. Many of the animals die in agony.

The Cruelty to Animals Act of 1876 contains six rules appertaining to experiments on animals, all excellent rules *if they were obeyed*, but they are not obeyed; experimenters can obtain exemption-certificates from the Home Office which exempt them from the rule about giving an animal an anaesthetic for painful experiments (and from three of the other rules, if exemption from these three rules is also desired). The National Antivivisection Society is hoping to get a Cruelty to Animals Act 1876 (Amendment) Bill passed before long. Mr Richard Body, MP, has indicated his willingness to introduce this Bill, which will abolish all exemption-certificates. The NAVS wants to bring about the total abolition of vivisection in the not-too-distant future, and will never be satisfied until this is accomplished. Meanwhile, the passing of an Amendment Bill abolishing all exemption-certificates will do a great deal to alleviate the sufferings of thousands of laboratory animals; indeed, there would be a drop in the number of animals used in any one year from about 5 million to less than one-quarter of a million.

There is really no possible justification for vivisection now that alternatives are available; moreover, alternatives that give more reliable results (the alternatives I have in mind are 'tissue' culture, diploid eggs, computers, unicellular organisms, etc), particulars of which can be obtained from 'FRAME', 312a Worple Road, Wimbledon, London SW20.

How many people realise, I wonder, that laboratory animals suffer so that Man may be relieved of *his* sufferings and may perhaps live a few years longer. But has Man the right to exploit animals so cruelly, in the hope of securing some possible (though doubtful) benefit for himself? In other words, can the practice of something that is ethically wrong ever be scientifically right? Surely the anser is 'No'.

The benefits believed to be derived from such experiments are very doubtful ones, for the simple reason that the resulting drugs, vaccines, etc, are, at best, merely palliative (they never cure anything) – at worst, they are dangerous because they tend to mask the early signs and symptoms of disease – to suppress Nature's warning signs. Also, owing to the fact that animals and humans are different species that differ physiologically, the testing of substances on animals is not a true and reliable guide as to whether or not they are suitable for giving to humans. The aforementioned alternative avenues of research do not conflict with humanitarian ideals, and if the time, money, and energy at present wasted on animal experimentation were devoted to these newer methods of research, everyone concerned would benefit, and medical research would make enormous strides forward.

For further reading, see *Crimes against Creation* compiled and published by Marie Dreyfus, 101 Hampden Road, London N8. *On Behalf of the Creatures*, by J. Todd-Ferrier, published by The Vegetarian Society, Parkdale, Dunham Road, Altrincham, Cheshire. *In Pity and in Anger* by John Vyvyan, published by Michael Joseph. *These We Have Not Loved* by V. A. Holmes-Gore, published by C. W. Daniel.

CHAPTER TEN

Ignorance
or Indifference?

How very seldom one sees, in the street or in a crowd, a face that one wants to look at twice – a face that is full of understanding and compassion. Of course, we are all at different stages of spiritual development, some people being more evolved (spiritually developed) than others. (This fact seems to provide some evidence for a belief in re-incarnation.) I suppose, therefore, that one ought to try to cultivate tolerance, though personally I find this difficult to do. The majority of people (I find) have so little imagination that they don't give a thought to how other living creatures live; they remain blissfully unaware of other peole's struggles and sufferings.

As for the sufferings of animals (other than domestic pets) these mean nothing to most people; yet they could help to reduce animal suffering in so many ways. For instance:
a) They could refrain from eating animal flesh. 'The fruits of the earth' are completely adequate substitutes for flesh foods; ideally, they should be eaten from the earth or the tree as soon as possible after they have been picked; it is best to eat them raw, as heat treatment (cooking) destroys much of their value, converting them from 'living' food into 'dead' food.

'Direct' feeding is the answer to the world food-shortage; to feed crops first to food-animals, and then eat the animal's flesh when it has been slaughtered, is a wasteful roundabout way of obtaining our nourishment. Likewise, plantmilk (made from soya beans) is another example of 'direct' feeding; it can and should replace cow's milk, the production of which involves so much suffering for the cow and her offspring, which are parted almost immediately after the birth of the offspring.

b) People could use soaps, creams, cosmetics, perfumes, etc, made from plant and flower substances rather than from whale-oil and other animal secretions, all of which are so cruelly obtained.

c) They could refrain from buying fur coats, calf-skin and snake-skin shoes and bags, sheepskin coats and boots, kid gloves, etc.

d) They could take herbal and biochemic remedies instead of doctors' drugs, the testing of which on animals involves such diabolical cruelty, as does the testing of cosmetics on animals too. For further information about experimentation on animals, see *The Dark Face of Science*, by John Vyvyan, published by Michael Joseph; also *Victims of Science* by Richard Ryder, published by Davis-Poynter. Cruelty-free cosmetics and soaps, etc, also simulation fur coats, can be obtained from BEAUTY WITHOUT CRUELTY, 40 High Street, Marylebone, London W1.

Public opinion is a very powerful weapon, and we (particularly housewives) could help to sharpen it, and make it more powerful still, by refusing to create a demand for cheap food, especially cheap flesh foods produced on factory-farms (I have in mind such things as broiler chicks, battery eggs, etc). For only with this weapon can we hope to defeat Public Enemy No. 1 – 'vested interests'. These (vested interests) are based on financial greed, and greed constitutes the greatest obstacle to Man's spiritual progress and enlightenment. It is greed that poisons Man's best intentions, and he will never be freed from the curse under which he is at present living so long as he exploits God's lesser creatures, the animals, and also the Earth on which he depends for food. (More about the rape of the Earth later.) He lives under the curse of ill-health (through unnatural feeding of his body), also the curse of being unable to live amicably and at peace with his fellow-creatures in all parts of the world. This inability to live peaceably without wars is also partly due to wrong feeding, because flesh foods stimulate the aggressive spirit in all who eat them.

'Man does not live by bread alone.' This is indisputably true. He has to be happy and to have a contented mind to be healthy, and he has to have a clear conscience to be happy (body and mind being so inter-dependent). But anyone who kills for food, or who tortures animals for knowledge, or who hunts them for clothing or for sport, such a person cannot, if he has a conscience, be happy and cannot, therefore, be healthy; neither can he who, although he may not actually commit these cruelties himself, condone them, and obtain what they produce, for his own use and consumption.

Man's inhumanity to Man is the direct outcome of his cruelty and injustice to animals, and so long as he continues to eat flesh foods there will always be wars. Ill-health and disease will continue too, for Man is not meant to eat the flesh of dead animals; his anatomy alone proves this. Carnivorous animals (i.e. flesh-eaters) have a short bowel, so that flesh-foods pass very quickly through their bodies and out of their gut. Man has a very long bowel, so that flesh foods pass very slowly through his gut, remaining much too long there, this time-lag causing them to putrefy (i.e. go rotten) and so to produce toxins which poison his bloodstream. Man became carnivorous during the first Ice Age when, because the Earth was covered with ice, he could get no vegetation to feed on, so he had to take to hunting wild animals for food. He has continued to hunt and to kill for food ever since, and has continued, as a consequence, to become less healthy. The fruits of the earth are his natural and, therefore, his best food.

CHAPTER ELEVEN

The Rape of the Earth

Man exploits the Earth, as well as animals. Present-day methods of farming and of agriculture aim at getting the last ounce of nourishment out of the soil, year after year, never resting it, green-manuring it, or putting back into it anything in the form of compost to replace the nourishment taken out of it by the crops. Artificial fertilisers are applied in order to produce bigger yields of crops (and therefore bigger bank-balances for the growers). But artificial fertilisers alone do not revitalise the soil; they simply flog it, acting like a whip used to flog a tired horse. Flogging it in this way year after year simply exhausts it, upsets its nice chemical balance, and destroys its living population (its earthworms, bacteria, and fungi), without which it is so much dead material. Thus, quality is sacrificed to quantity. But this sort of treatment cannot go on for ever; the time will come (indeed, it has already come) when Nature will hit back at Man for his greed.

For it *is* greed, not philanthropic motives, that prompts him to over-crop and over-graze the land, to cut down hedges between fields (despite the fact that hedges are the natural habitat of wild birds and that wild birds are natural predators and, therefore, Man's friends), and to poison the land with weed-killers and pesticides which destroy not only the weeds and the pests but also the creatures that feed on the pests.

Man also cuts down magnificent forests to provide grazing-ground for food-animals and wood-pulp for paper-making. If he but knew, this is suicidal, because, without trees, he would very soon die for want of oxygen. There would be no life on Earth if it were not for the presence of trees, which breathe out oxygen and breathe in carbon-dioxide. (This is the reverse of what we humans do; we breathe in oxygen and breathe out carbon-dioxide.)

If is, of course, the profit-motive that prompts these practices that rape the Earth. Such interference with Nature upsets the whole balance of Nature. Farmers try to justify their actions by pointing out that, owing to the population explosion, there would be a food shortage if they did not do these things. The answer to this is that there would be no food shortage, even in Eastern countries where there *is* a shortage at present, if people gave up eating flesh foods. Let me explain why:

It is estimated that 1½ acres of land that have been properly fertilised with composted organic matter will produce sufficient protein-rich crops to feed five people for one year, (such crops include cereals, nuts and seeds, pulses, etc), whereas the same sized piece of land will feed only one person for a year if it is used for growing crops to feed to food-animals which, after slaughter, are eaten by humans. This 'indirect' method of supplying protein-food to humans is a very wasteful, roundabout one, and, since the coming of factory-farming, huge supplies of grain (chiefly barley, and cotton-seed meal) are now required for the feeding of the factory-farm livestock. More than 370,000,000 tons of the world's grain harvest is fed annually to livestock – this is more than that consumed by all the humans in China and India put together. Thousands of tons of cotton-seed meal, to feed our food-animals, are imported annually from Eastern countries, thereby robbing the starving people of those countries of the food they grow to feed themselves. It is known that 10,000 human beings out East are dying of starvation every day, due to the wasteful methods of 'indirect' feeding practiced in Great Britain and other Western countries.

In the light of these facts, is it not our moral duty – quite apart from the fact that it is better for health reasons – to renounce flesh foods and become vegetarians (or vegans), so that the starving people of the world can have their fair share of what the bountiful Earth provides?

Some people may argue that a vegetarian diet (more especially a vegan diet which excludes milk, cheese, and eggs) *can* be deficient in 'complete' protein (the only sort of protein that is of any use to the body for body-building and body-maintenance). This is quite true. But to rectify this deficiency all that is required is a knowledge of how to combine 'incomplete' proteins in such a way as to form 'complete' proteins. Such knowledge can be acquired by reading 'How to be Healthy on a Vegetarian or Vegan Diet', in my book *Natural Remedies for Common Ailments* (published by C. W. Daniel, at £3·00).

CHAPTER TWELVE

To Tell You the Truth

Life teaches us many truths which, if they could be passed on to young travellers on life's road, might be very valuable to them. I will, therefore, try to pass on a few that I have learned, in the hope that other seekers after Truth will be helped thereby.

First, life has taught me that, in conformity with the law of KARMA (an ancient Eastern word for the natural law of 'Cause and Effect') we get the Fate we deserve – that we reap what we sow, and that *what* we are is the result of our own efforts (or lack of effort). In short, that *Character is Fate*.

'Ah,' you may say, 'but what about heredity? Do we not inherit our character and our constitution?' Yes, of course, up to a point we do; certainly the length of our earthly life depends to a great extent upon inherited vitality, but we do also make or mar our health and our happiness by our habits – our habits of eating, of thinking, and of living.

Our habits are, admittedly, tied up with, and influenced by, all the people with whom we come into daily contact, as well as by what we read, what we see, and what we hear. But these we *can* pick and choose to a very great extent, and thus we can mould our own character and our own fate. More especially we do so after our school-days are over, when we are freer to choose what we read, where we go, and with whom we associate.

The fact that we are very greatly influenced by the people with whom we come into contact is just another way of saying that we are all interdependent (the opposite of independent), that what people do, and think, and say, has a subtle influence on the lives and characters of other people; that each one of us is his brother's keeper; that Man's life is inextricably interwoven with the life and fate of all other living creatures, including birds, beasts, insects, trees, and plants; that all forms of life are complementary and interdependent.

Present-day scientific and agricultural research seems to entirely ignore or overlook 'ecology' (the interdependence of all living things). It produces chemical substances that upset the balance of Nature and the natural order of things; these include chemical fertilisers, poisonous sprays for killing pests and diseases on crops, stilboestrol and other sex hormones to stimulate growth and fat-production in food-animals. (These hormones make the animals *look* bigger and fatter, but do not increase their protein – only their fat, which is valueless.)

Many pest-controlling chemicals kill not only the pests themselves but the creatures that feed on the pests, thus doing more harm than good. They also poison bees that suck the honey from the plants and crops on which they are sprayed. These plants and crops are eaten by food-animals, and the animals and their produce (milk, butter, eggs, etc) are eaten by humans, who thus absorb a small dose of the chemical into *their* bodies (and, over a period of years, small doses mount up). Of course, some of these toxic chemicals can be, (and are) eliminated from the body, but some of them are cumulative poisons (i.e. poisons that build up in the body because they are never completely eliminated) and these eventually become a contributory cause of degenerative disease.

Artificial fertilisers upset the nice chemical balance of the soil; they also destroy earthworms and other valuable inhabitants of the soil, namely, bacteria and fungi. These tiny microscopic creatures, invisible to the naked eye, manufacture essential minerals out of decaying organic matter in the soil. These minerals dissolve in the soil-water, so long as it contains enough CO_2 (carbon-dioxide) to make it slightly acid; they would not otherwise dissolve in it, and they would then be unavailable to the plant. The CO_2 is produced by the fermentation of the decaying matter in the soil, so, if there *is* no decaying matter in the soil, no CO_2 is produced. This means that the soil-water is not rendered sufficiently acid to dissolve the essential minerals, and this means that the plant is deprived of its food. In other words, soil-water is not likely to be rich in minerals unless it is in contact with decaying matter which provides the CO_2 to make it slightly acid.

Thus it is apparent that it is simply futile to apply artificial fertilisers to the soil without at the same time applying decaying organic matter. (For further reading on the subject of the relationship between the soil population and plants, see that truly wonderful book by Lady Howard called *The Earth's Green Carpet*, published by Faber and Faber.)

It must be obvious to all intelligent people that only a healthy mineral-rich soil can produce healthy mineral-rich plants and, therefore, healthy animals and healthy humans; that, if the soil were properly treated, Man himself would not have to be treated (medically), and what a saving in national expenditure this would effect!

What is needed is a big educational campaign, particularly agricultural and nutritional education, in all schools, including medical training schools. The Government should recognise this need, and the medical profession should lead the campaign. As it is, National Health Service doctors continue to prescribe drugs and vaccines for the relief of what are really the early symptoms of 'deficiency' nutrition and incorrect feeding of the body. These drugs and vaccines are produced by scientists employed by big drug-companies, who are desirous only of making big incomes. They are a hindrance rather than a help to the body, opposing Nature's curative efforts. Moreover, they are tested and tried out on animals, such testing involving cruelty and suffering.

Man, by reason of his greater intelligence and therefore power, should regard himself as the Warden of the animal world, entrusted by the Almighty with the care and welfare of His little ones – as a nurse is entrusted by her employer with the care and welfare of his children.

D

Instead of which, Man exploits God's lesser creatures for his own material ends. He tortures them in the name of Science (nine-tenths of all laboratory experiments on animals are carried out without anaesthesia). He kills them for food. He shoots them for sport, sometimes simply wounding them and leaving them to die in agony. He chases them, and, if not caught and killed at the end of the chase, foxes often die of heart-disease due to exhaustion. Whales and seals are hunted by Man for their oils and their skins. The oils are used for soap-making, for cosmetics, and for making cooking-fats. Seal skins are made into fur coats.

Then there is the intensive exploitation of food-animals, as practised by modern factory-farming methods. (You can read all about the cruelty of these methods in a book called *Animal Machines* by Ruth Harrison, published by Faber and Faber.)

On these modern factory-farms the animals are treated as machines rather than as living sentient creatures. They are kept huddled together with barely enough room to stand, let alone move about. They spend their short lives in windowless sheds, in semi-darkness, deprived of sunlight, fresh air, exercise, and – in the case of calves – water. Their only function is to put on weight so that they will be ready for slaughter all the sooner. To hasten the process, they are given growth-stimulants, hormones, and tranquilisers, also antibiotics to suppress disease. At ten weeks old chickens are taken in crates (twelve birds to a crate) to the slaughterhouses of the packing-stations, having been starved for 16 hours before being packed. They remain in their crates sometimes for the best part of a day before their turn comes. They are then taken out of the crates, suspended upside down on a moving conveyor-belt, and, flapping wildly, each bird has its throat cut. Some packing-stations use mechanical stunners before throat-cutting (we have to thank the Humane Slaughter of Animals Association for this), other stations do not use it because the birds do not bleed properly if they are first stunned.

Veal calves and pigs are equally cruelly reared and slaughtered. Because the public demands white veal, the calves are kept tethered and confined in semi-darkness and are fed on a mineral-deficient diet devoid of roughage in order to make them anaemic. Water is withheld from them, so that, becoming desperately thirsty, they drink copiously of the synthetic milk-substitute which, together with growth-stimulants, hormones, etc, is given to them to make them fat.

The food-value of these animals – of pigs treated similarly, and of battery eggs – is very questionable. So, too, is the food-value of hens kept in batteries, and often dosed with pellets containing a dye for making the yolks of their eggs a deeper yellow. Such animals are certainly tasteless, and their flesh may even be detrimental to us as food.

Very soon, thanks to Mrs Joyce Butler's Labelling of Foods Bill, backed by the National Association for Health, of which anyone who wishes can become a member for as little as 50p a year, we hope that all factory-farm produce will be labelled as such; then housewives will have the option of refusing to buy such food. Meanwhile, we ask them to refrain from buying battery eggs, broiler chickens, veal, and pork, because, as everyone knows, demand creates supply.

The motive behind such inhumane methods of breeding and of rearing food-animals is not a philanthropic one – i.e. to feed the starving millions in the world. The motive is the profit motive, the get-rich-quick motive of big-business men. To feed the starving millions there is plenty of good vegetable-protein food available, enough for everybody, without killing animals for food, and there would be more if the grazing-land at present used for food-animals were used for crop-production. Moreover, such protein would be better and cleaner than flesh-foods, for these are full of the animals' waste-products and of all the drugs and vaccines with which the animals were dosed whilst they were alive. (See *Why kill for food?* by Geoffrey Rudd, published by The Vegetarian Society.)

For the same reason, Plantmilk (obtainable from most health-food shops now) is better food than cow's milk, much of which contains hormones and antibiotics with which cows are injected. *Granogen*, a soya-bean milk-food, is an almost complete food. It is a product of vegetarian nutritional research which differs from other forms of scientific research in that it involves no experiments on animals. Such research deserves all the support we can give it.

Other diabolically cruel practices that Man pursues are blood-sports, the keeping of wild animals and birds in cages (tame ones too, like rabbits), and the training of circus animals to perform in public.

These practices, together with those already mentioned – i.e. vivisection, the slaughter of animals and birds for food, the hunting and killing of wild animals and of whales and seals for their skins and oils, the torture of civet cats for their secretions, the forcible feeding of geese to increase the size of their livers – these are only a few of the many practices in which Man exploits animals for his own profit and pleasure.

Actually, as far as vivisection is concerned, this form of exploitation does *not* benefit Man. It is a futile waste of time and money to experiment on animals for the purpose of finding out how to treat disease in Man, for the simple reason that animals and humans are different species, and so they react differently to the various drugs, etc, that enter their blood-streams.

Professor Voronoff, the eminent scientist, said that if a cure for cancer were ever discovered as the result of experiments on rats, it would cure cancer in rats, but not in humans. It was also noticed by another eminent scientist, Dr Rowe Hall, that English mice that had been inoculated against cancer and then injected with cancer cells, could be protected against the disease to an extent of 90 per cent, whereas only 10 per cent of *Danish* mice, which were used under exactly the same conditions, survived. If there is such a difference between the reactions of different breeds of mice, there must be an even greater difference between the reactions of mice and of men.

Vaccination against smallpox is another outcome of experiments on animals; so, too, is inoculation with antitoxin against diphtheria, and inoculation with insulin for diabetes. Statistics refute the claims made by experimenters that these substances have reduced the risk of infection and death from smallpox,

To Tell You the Truth

diphtheria, and diabetes. Statistics have proved what a failure they have all been. These statistics can be obtained from the Anti-vaccination Society, 2a Lebanon Road, Croydon, Surrey.

For instance, there was a great epidemic of smallpox in Great Britain, the greatest on record – in 1870–71, when over 42,000 people died of the disease, despite the fact that practically the whole population had been vaccinated.

As for diphtheria, the death-rate rose steadily for five years after the introduction of the diphtheria-anti-toxin treatment, while at the same time the death-rate from other infectious diseases fell, due of course, to improved conditions of sanitation and hygiene. From this it can be inferred that, but for the anti-toxin, the diphtheria death-rate would have fallen also.

The death-rate for diabetes has gone on steadily rising ever since the introduction of insulin treatment; this statement can be verified by statistics. (See *The Hazards of Immunisation* by Sir Graham Wilson.)

Thus we see the futility of trying to prevent disease by inoculation, to say nothing of the cruelty involved in the experiments on animals in order to obtain the inoculation-substances. All these things – drugs, inoculations, serums, vaccines, etc, all of which are tested and tried out on animals, have been unsuccessful in curing any of the commoner present-day diseases from which Man suffers – such things as cancer, diabetes, coronary thrombosis, etc; indeed, they very often cause a worsening of the patient's condition, and hasten his death.

The soundness and rightness of a method or practice can be judged only by allowing one's conscience to be the judge of its soundness and rightness. *'Science, without Conscience, is but death of the Soul', wrote Montaigne.* The late Lord Chief Justice Coleridge said *'There is no such thing as necessary cruelty, any more than there is necessary sin'.*

The basis of morality is Compassion, and the Church, which is a body of people who represent morality, should make a stand against all such cruel and therefore immoral practices. The Church should take the lead and, by disclosing the horrifying facts, try to influence people to abandon the practices, and to live in closer co-operation with Nature. As it is, most clergymen, after Sunday service, sit down happily, like millions of other people, to a dinner of dead animal or bird, deliberately shutting out from their minds all thought of what the procuring of such food has entailed, in suffering, for the animal, and in degradation for the slaughterman. In this respect, like most people, they lack imagination, which has been aptly described as 'the ability to face facts'.

We pride ourselves on being civilised and a nation of animal-lovers, but is it civilised to lavish affection and care upon one species of animal (our pets) and to kill and eat another species (food-animals)? It is certainly inconsistent so to do.

The vast majority of people have silenced 'the still, small voice of Conscience', and have hardened their hearts and minds because of their palate's desire for the taste of flesh-foods and flesh-food delicacies. Do you think we have any right to create a demand for flesh food, simply in order to satisfy our desire for the taste of it? The demand creates the supply, let us remember.

We eat to live, not vice-versa, and flesh-foods are not necessary items of food; indeed, some flesh foods such as pork, bacon, ham, pork sausages, etc, are sometimes actually diseased, and people can become diseased through eating them. Trichinosis, a most horrible disease, is very common in pigs, and it can be transmitted to the eater of pig-meat. So, also, can tuberculosis and other diseases. Even *healthy* flesh-foods cause an accumulation of acid waste-products in the human body, which, through incomplete elimination of them, can and do cause disease.

But bodily disease is not the only consequence of eating flesh-foods; Man's mind and spirit are adversely affected thereby, for flesh-foods not only poison his blood but make him aggressive and foster a war-like spirit in him. It is possible that there would be no crime-waves or wars, and far fewer criminals of every sort, if Man gave up eating dead animals. The eating of flesh-foods is a self-inflicted curse under which Man is living, a curse which is adversely affecting not only his health, peace of mind, and his happiness, but which is fast robbing the Earth of its green carpet and its trees (without which all life on Earth would cease). Magnificent trees are continually being cut down in order to make space for more grazing-land for food-animals, and to provide the wood-pulp for paper-making. (Much of the paper is used for newpaper, on which is printed news of Man's crimes, quarrels, greed, and other horrors.)

The rape of the Earth is the direct result of Man's love of flesh-foods and of money. The Sahara desert is the result of a cutting-down of the forest, and of its vegetation having been cropped bare by food-animals. In New Zealand, South Africa, and Australia, sheep have eaten all the green undergrowth. In fact, land-erosion due to over-grazing is world-wide, and unless the vicious circle of more stock-breeding, more grazing, and consequently more land-erosion, is broken, Man cannot survive much longer. In view of the population-explosion, his only hope of survival is the adoption of a fleshless diet.

The wanton destruction of magnificent forests, the over-grazing of the land by food-animals, the over-cropping of the land for commercial gain – these are the underlying causes of present-day Man's sickness of body and of soul. He is a slave to his palate, and ruled by his love of money. These obsessions constitute the greatest obstacles to his spiritual progress. They poison his best intentions, thus marring his happiness.

Man will never know true happiness and peace of mind – nor real wealth, (for wealth cannot be measured in terms of money or possessions) so long as he continues to exploit God's lesser creatures to satisfy his carnal appetites, and to rape the good Earth for the sake of financial gain.

CHAPTER THIRTEEN

Knowledge and Wisdom

We are very 'education-conscious' nowadays, and rightly so if it is education in its widest sense that is provided; but so often education seems to be confused with book-learning, which is something quite different. School education consists largely of this, and of memory-training. These are useful branches of education but they do not constitute its main trunk, and they should not be allowed to obscure its real object, which is to stimulate a desire for knowledge in its widest sense; this includes knowledge of all the wonders and beauties of Nature and of Art; knowledge of great men and women and of what they achieved; knowledge of how the human body works and of what its needs are; knowledge of soil-science and of how to produce nutritionally-rich food-crops; knowledge of other crafts, such as bee-keeping, bread-making, etc.

A knowledge of the above is surely of far greater interest and importance than dry-as-dust book-learning and memory-training.

Every child over the age of 12 should receive instruction at school in elementary anatomy and physiology; in correct feeding and in the correct preparation of foods (cooked *and* raw); in correct breathing, and in Dr Alexander's methods of conserving energy through economy of effort (see *Conservation of Energy*, chapter three). The instruction could take the form of a weekly (or bi-weekly) lecture by a visiting Naturopath who, unlike a member of the orthodox medical profession, will have received training in correct feeding, etc. There should be a lending-library of books on 'health' subjects in the school, and the children should be advised by the Naturopath of suitable ones to read.

It is because of the lack of 'health' education that there is so much unnecessary ill-health and suffering in the world. Much of this could be avoided if people understood the needs of their bodies, and how best to meet those needs. It is ignorance and apathy – *and* misplaced faith in the power of the doctor to cure – that is at the root of much illness and disease, so that our hospitals are full to overflowing. A belief in the power of the doctor to cure what is very often the result of incorrect feeding is the biggest obstacle between man and his good health. Too late he realises that the doctor *cannot* cure him; that prevention, by means of right eating, right thinking, and right living, is the only sure cure.

But to return to the subject of education. The born educator is one who can present a subject to his pupils in such a way as to arouse in them a keen desire to learn, and to go on learning. He is an educator in the real sense of the word. He stimulates in his pupils a *desire* for knowledge. This is the first essential; the *acquisition* of knowledge will follow automatically.

Knowledge, of course, is not at all the same thing as Wisdom. Wisdom is not tested by the schools; it cannot be passed from one possessing it to one not possessing it, because, as Walt Whitman said, 'Wisdom is of the Soul'. Highly-evolved people are born with wisdom. Others are not born with it, but they are born with a desire to acquire it, and with the necessary courage and endurance for the long struggle which the acquisition of it entails.

Thousands of people have great brain-power and are well-educated in the book-learning sense, but often these people lack wisdom. This is really because they fail to recognise Truth when they meet it. As Sir Winston Churchill once said – 'Men occasionally stumble over the Truth, but usually they do not examine it; they pick themselves up and hurry off, as if nothing had happened.'

Most people close their minds early in life and become unreceptive to the influence and ideas of people and of books, etc, with which they come into contact. They stumble over Truth many times, but fail to recognise it. They get 'set' in their habits and beliefs, and so they never acquire wisdom – nor, I believe, deep happiness. The minds of children are malleable, and they can be taught correct feeding of the body, and correct utilisation of their vital forces; as well as how to think right, and how to appreciate the Eternal Verities. But for this they require the right kind of teachers, *and* parents. Simple country folk who live close to Nature, whose natural inborn wisdom has not been blunted by contact with civilisation (so-called), are often some of the wisest and godliest of people. Their book-learning may be scanty, but they possess an intuitive wisdom which guides them throughout their lives, enabling them to obey Nature's laws, and therefore to enjoy a healthy, long and happy life.

CHAPTER FOURTEEN

The Divine Purpose

It seems to me that the sole purpose of our sojourn here on Earth – the Divine Purpose, if you like – is the development of our souls. As we develop, the people who come into contact with us may be helped and influenced beneficially by us, just as we, in our turn, can be helped and influenced by other developing souls. The capacity to absorb and profit by other people's spoken and written words varies in each one of us; some people are much more sensitive and receptive than others; the capacity to profit by experience also varies. This being so, it follows that 'Experience' (*per se*) is of no value; if it were, the paving stones of London would be wiser than its wisest men. And, of course, it is not only the written and the spoken word that exercise an influence (and contribute to) the development of the soul. The influence of example is a subtle (below the-surface) one, but very powerful; this is the influence exerted by the way we conduct ourselves, the way we behave, and the way we speak and look.

The influence of Mind over Mind is the means whereby the Divine Purpose is being achieved. When this purpose (the development of men's souls) has been achieved, the Brotherhood of Man will be a reality and there will be peace on Earth. Meanwhile, we struggle and suffer, and live and learn, thus contributing to the achievement of the Divine Purpose and the coming of a 'Golden Age'. Civilisation, which, in many ways, is so *un*civilised, hinders rather than helps the Divine Purpose.

For example, the eating of unnatural foods (including the flesh of dead animals, birds, and fishes) is the result of civilisation and the discovery of fire for cooking such foods. Until the discovery of fire, primitive Man lived on the fruits of the Earth and of the trees (seeds, nuts, fruits, leaves and shoots, and probably grasses) and these are therefore his natural foods. Flesh foods and all other cooked foods are unnatural foods and detrimental to health (physical *and* mental); thus the physiological result of a civilised diet has been the insurgence of disease and of psychosomatic disorders. The explanation is as follows.

All living things, including plants, animals, and Man, need sustenance for the building and maintenance of their bodies. This sustenance has to be re-organised by the body before it can become part of the body-structure. (In the case of plants, it is converted into plant-structure by the sun's energy). Digestion of food in Man is a coming-to-terms with it, a re-organising of it into body-substance, a mysterious spiritualising process, not really understood. The way food is re-organised by Man is quite different from the way it is re-organised by an animal. To eat dead animals and their organs is therefore an unwise thing to do, and places a great burden on the human body. It is also a dangerous thing to do, as animals are unnaturally reared (*and* fed) nowadays, and often riddled with disease. The vibration rate of their cells is also different from the vibration rate of human cells, and to eat their flesh and their products is therefore of doubtful benefit, indeed, it is thought by some nutritionists to be detrimental to human health.

But, apart from the health angle, there is the ethical point of view. It is difficult to understand how otherwise likeable, kindly people can, by eating flesh foods, condone the diabolical cruelty of killing animals for food. Demand for a substance creates supply, and so, until people can be persuaded to abandon meat-eating, the supply will continue. I believe the demand would soon cease altogether if people could go and see what goes on inside a slaughter-house, and if they were then asked whether they would still eat meat if they had to do the killing of it themselves, most of them would indignantly reply 'No. I would not'.

'Then what right have you to expect someone else to do such brutalising work *for* you?' you could ask them. The answer is, of course, 'No right'. High wages paid to slaughter-men do not make up for the degradation of such diabolical work.

CHAPTER FIFTEEN

Flesh Foods, Are They Necessary?

Testimonies to the fact that they are not.
'It is a vulgar error to regard meat in any form as necessary to life. All that is necessary to the human body can be supplied by the vegetable kingdom.

It is a fact beyond all question that people who live on vegetarian food are stronger and healthier, and that the prevailing meat diet is not only a wasteful extravagance but a source of serious evil to the consumer.

I am compelled by facts to accept the conclusion that more physical evil accrues to Man from erroneous habits of diet than from alcoholic drink.'

(Sir Henry Thompson, MD, FRCS in 'Food and Feeding')

'Flesh food is material that has been rendered toxic during the animal's lifetime. In the first place, his endocrine defences are interfered with by castration. He is then immobilised and overfed, with a view to causing him to develop fatty-degeneration of all his organs; and it is when this ugly process is complete that he is regarded as fit for human consumption.'

(Dr Leonard Williams in 'The Practitioner')

'No physiologist would dispute the fact that Man's natural diet is a vegetable one.'

(Dr Spenser Thompson)

'Flesh eating is not necessary to health.'
(*'Encyclopaedia Britannica 1973'*)

'It is impossible to challenge the statement that the human body can be properly nourished on a vegetarian diet. Research has established a sound scientific basis for the belief that Man can live healthily without flesh foods.'
(*Stated by Sir Jack Drummond, wartime adviser to the Ministry of Health*)

'It is immaterial whether the protein units are derived from plant or from animal foods. There is no evidence that animal-protein has any intrinsic value of its own.'
(*Stated by the Nutrition Committee of the British Medical Association*)

'Undeniably it is more natural to live on a vegetarian diet.'
(*The Family Health Encyclopaedia, Mind and Body, published by Orbis Publishing Company*)

'Nutritionally, vegetable substances possess the most striking advantages over flesh foods. I should like to see the vegetable-and-fruit diet in more general use, and I believe it will be.'
(*Sir Benjamin Richardson*, MD, FRS)

'It is clear that the proteins of cereals, roots, and leafy vegetables provide an excellent blend of all the essential amino-acids (building-blocks) needed for body-tissue construction and body-maintenance.'
(*Sir Jack Drummond, late Professor of Biochemistry, University of London*)

'Flesh foods are not the best nourishment for humans, and were not eaten by our primitive ancestors.'
(*Dr J. H. Kellogg*, MD)

'There are many alternative sources of first-class protein, and a meatless diet is as good as any other.'
(*Lord Hill of Luton*, MD, DPH, LLD)

Flesh foods, are they detrimental to health?

The late Mr Kasper Blond, FRCS, eminent cancer specialist and author of *Liver Damage as a Cause of Cancer*, believed that cancer is a degeneration of body-tissue caused by damage to the liver by long years of faulty feeding on flesh foods, and of incomplete elimination of waste-products from the body. He condemned the eating of flesh foods because, he said, they are never *completely* digested, and the undigested portions go rotten in the large bowel and produce poisons damaging to the liver. He writes 'Man is the only animal who cooks food before eating it. It is likely that cooking renders meat unsuitable for assimilation because it destroys its vitamins and enzymes, and these are essential to its digestion and assimilation. The prevention of liver damage is the main problem; the other problem is the regeneration of an already damaged liver. I am *convinced* that a diet free from animal protein is the most important factor in such regeneration.'

Other eminent doctors who have also advised the omission of flesh foods from everyone's diet include the following:

Dr Szekely author of *Medicine Tomorrow*

Dr Bircher-Benner, MD author of *The Prevention of Incurable Disease*

Dr Maud Fere, LRCPS, DPH author of *Cancer, Its Dietetic Cause and Cure*

Dr W. H. Hay, MD author of *Health via Food*

Dr Hauschka, DSC author of *Nutrition*

Dr Vogel author of *The Nature Doctor*

Dr Roger Williams, MD author of *Nutrition Against Disease*

Flesh foods, the production of which is so barbarous, are they destructive of peace of mind, of a guilt-free conscience, and therefore of sound health?

Testimonies to the fact that they *are* unethical and harmful, not only to physical health but also to mental health and peace of mind, are legion, and can be found in the following books by eminent writers, past and present:

The Ethics of Diet by Howard Williams, MA

Vindication of a Natural Diet by Percy Bysshe Shelley

The Philosophy of Compassion by Esme Wynne Tyson

The First Step (from *Essays*) by Count Leo Tolstoi

On Abstinence From Animal Food by Prophry (Centaur Press)

On Behalf of the Creatures by The Rev Todd Ferrier

The Rights of Animals by Brigid Brophy (*Sunday Times* article)

Animal Machines by Ruth Harrison

Why Kill For Food? by Geoffrey Rudd (The Vegetarian Society)

The Holy Bible (Genesis IX, 4)
'But flesh, with the life thereof, which is the blood thereof, shall ye not eat'

Food for a Future by Jon Wynne Tyson

*Food for the Golden Age** by Frank Wilson

*Food Fit for Humans** by Frank Wilson

The Basis of Morality by Schopenhauer

*The Recovery of Culture** by Henry Bailey Stevens

* The C. W. Daniel Co, London

CHAPTER SIXTEEN

Our Social System Today

What we need, and what I'm afraid we shall never get, is a social system based on freedom, freedom of every kind. We shall never get it because instinctively we know that it wouldn't work, that the vast majority of people would abuse it, and that the result would be complete and utter chaos.

Yet people *need* freedom – freedom from the day-to-day slavery of having to do jobs they dislike in order to earn enough money to buy the necessities of life; – perhaps not *complete* freedom, but certainly *more* freedom, to be used for the refreshment of the spirit and the resting of the Psyche (the Personality) which, just as the physical body needs sleep, needs rest and relaxation. Sensuous pleasures, which allow Man to divest himself of his Personality – to throw it off as he throws off his garments – are most essential to the well-being of his body, mind, and spirit. These pleasures include the pleasure of sexual intercourse with a loved one, the pleasure of listening to beautiful music, the pleasure of contemplating the wonders and beauties of Nature and of Art, and the pleasure of using the body muscles in games and sports requiring skill.

Unfortunately, the masses have little time or opportunity for any of these pleasures other than the pleasure of sexual intercourse, and, even if they *had*, they are generally incapable of deriving sufficient pleasure from them to make them beneficially relaxing. However, it is doubtful that they can be *helped* to increase their pleasure in the spiritual and intellectual pleasures of great music, the wonders and beauties of Nature and of Art, etc, because love of these things is probably inborn, cultivatable only if it already exists in embryo inside us.

What is needed for the masses is education in the widest sense of the word – education in 'the Humanities', in Ecology, in the Arts, and in the crafts that enable them to be self-supporting, rather than in Science and Technology.

Man's spiritual development has certainly not kept pace with his intellectual development. His achievements in Science and Technology have been prodigious, but they have been at the expense of his soul. As a consequence, he is no healthier or happier as a result of them; neither does he live longer – indeed, he does not live as long as his early ancestors; this is largely because he eats unnatural food (cooked flesh foods and other cooked or processed foods). It seems pretty certain therefore that, unless and until Man's spiritual development catches up with his brain development, and unless and until he re-learns to eat only natural foods (unnatural foods hinder spiritual development), he will never enjoy true health of mind or body, even though he may acquire more freedom. As Sir Arthur Conan Doyle so wisely said,

'The greatest danger that can come to a nation is that its intellect should outrun its soul. This was the cause of the downfall of Atlantis, and of all the other great Powers.'

CHAPTER SEVENTEEN

Passing the Time

You often hear people say – referring perhaps to television, or to films, or to card-playing, or some other game – 'It helps to pass the time.'

But why, in Heaven's name, should anyone *want* simply to pass the time? Surely time goes by all too quickly, and is just the one thing that we want more of. With a longer time on Earth we could solve (and help others to solve) many more of the problems and difficulties that Mankind has to tackle. To gain more time on Earth, we *must* retain (or regain, if lost) good health. That makes health of more importance than anything else, for without it we can be of no use to ourselves, or to Mankind.

There is an old Latin proverb which says 'Learn first how to live, and then philosophise'. In other words, it is essential to first learn the art of living a healthy natural life; for if we are sick, or if we die at an early age, of what use are we to society? We cannot help to solve the problems that society has to face; we cannot even solve our own problems with equanimity and a calm mind (body and mind being so closely interrelated and interdependent). Moreover, we cannot enjoy life to the full, and of what use is it, therefore, to be gifted or clever (or both) if our health won't allow us to enjoy life? So, learn first how to live; then you will live longer, and gain more time for philosophising, for helping others, and for enjoying life.

Regarding the subject of pastimes, a purely 'passive' use of *some* of the precious hours of our all-too-short earthly life is, of course, a salutary thing; for to do, to look at, and to hear things that give us pleasure, provides rest and refreshment for the mind (and therefore benefits the body).

Unfortunately, though, many pastimes just *dope* the mind instead of stimulating, diverting, and entertaining it. It is thus that many elderly and invalid people, no longer able to fill their days with activities, yet still capable of using their mental powers if not their muscles, allow their minds to atrophy with disuse. They indulge in too much passive and not enough active (self-produced) entertainment.

By self-produced entertainment, I mean the making of something, either with hands or brain (or both). For instance, the writing of a story, or the playing of a musical instrument, or the painting of a picture, or the making of a garment, or the weaving of a material or rug, or the construction of something – there are dozens of creative pastimes with which we can provide our own entertainment. Of course, a little of the passive 'push-button' type of entertainment, which we sit back and enjoy with our eyes or ears, is salutory and beneficial to mind and body; but this sort of passive entertainment should not be indulged in to the exclusion of the active self-made sort. A little of each sort is what we really need.

Creative people are undoubtedly the happiest people. Next happiest are the people who are not themselves creative, but who can appreciate the beautiful and worth-while creations of other people, great books, great music, great art, etc.

Least happy are the people who can neither create nor appreciate the great creations of others. They desire only that their thoughts should be diverted from themselves and their surroundings; that they should be 'taken out of themselves' and made to forget, allowed to escape from, the realities of life. These are the people who lack an inner peace and a tranquility of spirit. These are the people (and they come from all age-groups) who talk about doing things 'to pass the time', and they are to be pitied, because they must be the least happy of mortals. If only they could be made to realise that happiness comes from within, because God dwells within. It is doubtful whether talking to them would help them to realise it; example might, if they are lucky enough to come into contact with someone who *does* realise it, and *is* a living example of it.

CHAPTER EIGHTEEN

The Answer
to Loneliness

Sometimes, people say to me 'I wonder you don't have a cat or dog to keep you company; you must be very lonely, living alone'. But being alone and being lonely are two quite different things. People are not necessarily lonely who have neither human nor animal company. Conversely, people who have both kinds of company *are* very often lonely, because loneliness is really a state of mind. It is an empty bored state of mind; this means that one can feel lonely, irrespective of whether or not one *is* alone.

In all the important things of life we *are* alone, of course, in spirit if not in body. It is only in superficial ways that we can make contact with other people; the things of the spirit we can hardly ever share. As Aldous Huxley said, we are each one of us serving a life-sentence of solitary confinement. This is true of the vast majority of people; the lucky few who have found a kindred spirit with whom to share life need help and comfort only when they have lost their 'good companion'.

First, then, it is well to realise that nearly everyone is as lonely in spirit as everyone else; that, for the vast majority of people, loneliness is inevitable.

The next thing to realise is that loneliness need not be the dreadful thing it is usually considered to be, because, by achievement, we can turn it from a barren negative state into a positive productive one. To do this will take time, and will entail patience and perseverance, but it *can* be done – I know it can, because I have done it. I did it by reading books on one particular subject in which I felt a deep interest and about which I desired to know more, and, if *I* can do it, so can you – provided you have your eyesight (see note * at the end of this chapter).

Anyone with intelligence, and the desire to learn *can* learn anything and everything nowadays. Wonderful books on every subject are available from public libraries everywhere, and, if you don't know which books to ask for, the Head Librarian is always very pleased to help and advise you to get the books you need (again I speak from experience).

Loneliness, especially of older people, is said to be one of the major social problems of our day and age. Old people's clubs, outings, socials, visits from social workers, all these efforts of kindly people treat the symptoms but not the cause of the loneliness. I believe the cause is very often simply boredom, due to mind starvation, and that, like many bodily ailments, it is self-curable by means of 'selective' feeding with the right foods, i.e. with 'food for thought'.

I believe, however, that books and book-learning are only a means to an end; that learning, by itself, does not necessarily bring either happiness or wisdom, because a man can be learned yet not wise. Wisdom does not come from learning, but from intuition and experience. What *does* come from learning is knowledge, and knowledge enables Man to create – with his brain or with his hands, or with both – and thus to give expression to his personality, and thereby fulfil his strongest urge. Moreover, once he is able to create, he produces something that mirrors his personality, and this reflection of himself banishes loneliness.

First and foremost, therefore, in order to change your barren negative state of loneliness into a positive productive one, you need a thirst for knowledge – for general knowledge, to start with. This will gradually narrow down to a thirst for knowledge of one particular subject. Reading romances and thrillers, which are simply dope, will not cure your loneliness. I started off on my search for knowledge as a cure for loneliness by reading a book called *Your Daily-Bread* by Doris Grant. Reading this book led to reading others on the all-important subject of nutrition in relation to health, and gradually I acquired a vast store of knowledge on the subject, which I set down in my book *Handbook of Health*.

Maybe you are not the sort of person who likes making things with your hands, or you may be the sort that couldn't care less about what you eat and drink (though I hope you are not, because what you eat and drink can make or mar your health). In this case, books on 'crafts' or on Nutrition will not appeal to you, and a book on some other subject will be the right one to start you off on the road to knowledge. Each one of us is different, with differing likes and dislikes, differing abilities and ambitions, and only you yourself can discover (through dipping into this and that book, till you find one that holds your attention and interest), what line is *your* particular line.

Having acquired a thirst for knowledge, you need leisure and time for reading, for digesting what you have read, and for meditation (which is another name for prayer). Being alone, you *have* all these things, and many people, who are continually surrounded by other people, would envy you and your 'aloneness' and the golden opportunities it affords for reading and for quiet meditation. These people – the people who are never alone – are not likely to have enough leisure, time, or peace for the pursuit of knowledge and the power of self-expression that it brings.

The people who *are* alone are free to read, to think, to meditate, and to develop spiritually; they can make books their friends and companions, and what better friends and companions can anyone want? Books are silent friends, yet they speak *volumes*!

Other people who are alone but not lonely are the people who have found what can only be described as 'the way, the truth and the light'. They are not lonely because they are aware of God's company, and this fills them with a warm and comforting sense of companionship. They have come to realise that God is an all-pervading power-for-good; that a tiny fraction of that power is to be found to a greater or lesser degree in everyone; that God is not external to anyone or anything, nor in one certain place, but is present wherever and whenever anyone feels a need for God's presence. God is a living reality to these people, an ever-present source of strength and of companionship. They are often the loneliest people in the worldly sense, but the least lonely in the spiritual sense. They enjoy being alone with their thoughts, their books, their hobbies, and with Nature. They understand the words of R. L. Stevenson, who said:

> The world is so full of a number of things,
> I think we should all be as happy as kings.

How these people have acquired this inner peace and happiness cannot be explained in words. Each one of us has to grope about and discover Truth (another name for God) for himself. There is no royal road to success, nor any guarantee that you will reach the end of the road, but the chances are that you *will*, if your desire to do so is strong enough. Also, it is wonderful how help seems to pour in from all directions, once you get started. You meet people now and then whose actions and reactions, whose kindness and courtesy, whose whole way of living, teaches you much, and helps your progress along the road to Truth. Admittedly, we don't meet many such people, but we do all meet a few, I think.

Of course, it helps if we also have what I can only describe as 'a nose for Truth' – a sort of inherent ability to 'nose' it out. This is because, like a buried bone which a dog, through his sense of smell, can find, Truth has to be tracked down and unearthed. Bit by bit you find it, and gradually the bits fit together like a jig-saw puzzle, until at last the whole wonderful picture takes shape, and Truth becomes clear to you.

All lonely people should regard loneliness as the price they have to pay for freedom to develop spiritually and to find Truth. In time, they will come to realise that what they gain is worth the price they have to pay.

*NB.   If any of my readers have poor eyesight and find reading tiring, even with glasses, they should read, or get someone to read to them – a book called *Better sight without glasses* by Harry Benjamin, published by Health for All, Beaver House, York Close, Byfleet, Weybridge, Surrey. It contains helpful advice and eye exercises. The author, a Nature-cure practitioner, cured himself of threatened blindness when orthodox doctors had given up hope of saving his sight. They should also eat foods rich in Vitamin A (see my book *Handbook of Health*, published by Mayflower Books); drink home-made sage tea, and use Potter's *Eyebright* eye-lotion.

CHAPTER NINETEEN

Biochemic Therapy and Psionic Medicine

How often one meets people who are tired, listless, or depressed. Then, when you hear that they are 'under the doctor' and having drugs of one sort or another for this or that ailment, you are only surprised that their tiredness, depression, etc, is not worse than it is. Truly, the human body is wonderfully adaptable and 'tough', but drug-happy doctors (and most of them *are* nowadays) should be reminded that the amount of ill-treatment the human body will stand (in the form of corrective drugs) *is* limited; that corrective drugs simply suppress the symptoms, which are Nature's warnings and which should be heeded, *not* suppressed; that drugs give a false sense of security, by misleading the patient into thinking that they have remedied the cause of the symptoms, whereas in reality no attempt has been made to *find* the cause.

And how little interest many NHS doctors take in their patients. The case of an elderly widow comes to mind, whose medical history is as follows:

25 years ago – Hysterectomy operation.

6 years ago – Gall-bladder removed.

4 or 5 years ago – Four toes on each foot removed because of Arthritis.

6 months ago – A heart attack.

Now she has an ulcerated mouth and soft palate, gets into a panic in case she is unable to swallow, and suffers from lack of appetite and great depression. Yet her doctor had never mentioned diet, she said; nor had he questioned her about her digestion or her bowel movements, nor prescribed anything other than digitalis pills and nerve-sedative tablets. Moreover, despite the fact that she is over 70 and walks with pain and great difficulty, she has to walk to his surgery if she wants to see him (she has no car and he never offers to go and see her at her house), and, after waiting sometimes nearly an hour to see him, the interview lasts usually only five minutes, or less. She is only one of many people who all tell the same story, from which it is clear that doctors do not concern themselves with their patients' diets, nor their way of life; they seem concerned only with suppressing symptoms with corrective drugs, and always the drug is digitalis for *all* heart troubles, bismuth or bicarbonate of soda for digestive troubles, aspirin for pain, pheno-barbitone for 'nerves', and salicylate of soda for rheumatic troubles. Their drug repertory seems to be very limited, in fact, I understand that, under the rules of the National Health Service, doctors are not allowed to prescribe remedies other than those listed on the 'permitted' list. This list does *not* include Biochemic remedies yet Biochemic remedies have been proved to be very beneficial, and have cured many ailments that orthodox medicine could do nothing for. Unlike corrective drugs, Biochemic remedies are all substances (minerals and trace-elements) that enter into the composition of the cells and tissues of the body. According to Dr Gilbert and other Biochemic doctors, a deficiency of one or more of these mineral substances ('tissue salts' they are called) is the real cause of most bodily disorders (physical *and* mental).

A brief explanation of the principles of Biochemic therapy is as follows. In normal health, the food we eat should supply us (provided it is grown in fertile composted soil) with all the nutrients, minerals, and trace-elements our body cells require. The minerals and trace-elements are carried by the blood, together with food-nutrients, water, and oxygen, to all the cells and tissues of the body, and they play a vital part in the building-up and the breaking-down processes of the body cells. Indeed, without them, all cell-activity – all growth, repair-work, all heat and energy production, in other words, all life – would cease, because the body cells can absorb and combine with food nutrients only in the presence of certain minerals and trace-elements. When the food nutrients are deficient in (or under-supplied with) these essential minerals and trace-elements, cell activity slows down, gradually the cells lose their power of absorption, and symptoms of bodily disorder and ill-health follow. The cells then become too weak to make use of even food containing all the essential nutrients *and* minerals; they are so weak that they need *finer* particles of minerals than those normally found in food. In other words, when a deficiency reaches the point where illness occurs, the deficiency cannot be made good by food, not even by good food. This is where Biochemic therapy steps in and comes to the rescue. A Bio-chemic remedy supplies the necessary mineral or trace-element (the one that the symptoms indicate is missing) in a form in which it can be directly absorbed into the bloodstream. This mineral or trace-element is split up into minute molecules (the process is called 'trituration') which are dispersed in lactose and then moulded into tiny pills. The dose (two or three of the pills) is allowed to dissolve *very* slowly in the mouth, and thus the minute particles are absorbed directly into the bloodstream through the tiny blood-vessels (the capillaries) in the lining of the mouth, throat, and gullet. They never reach the stomach, where the acid of the gastric juices would change them chemi-cally. Thus they reach the body-cells in a finely-triturated, chemically-unchanged form – a form in which they can be most easily assimilated by the weakened cells. For example, in anaemic people, the body cells indicate (by the symptoms) a lack of iron; but it is very often useless to give these people a diet rich in iron-containing foods, because, when the foods are eaten, the iron in them is changed chemically (by the hydro-chloric acid in the gastric juices) into chloride of iron, which is *not* the form of iron the cells are crying out for. The form of iron needed is best obtained from biochemic ferro-phosphate pills, which are allowed to dissolve slowly in the mouth.

Moreover, as Biochemic remedies are so finely triturated, and thus can be absorbed directly into the bloodstream through the walls of the mouth and throat without having to pass through the stomach, they are a form of treatment which is not affected by the digestive and absorptive disability which so often accompanies illness. (For further information see *The Earthy Basis of Health* by Dr Peter Gilbert of 42 Harley Street, London W1. Also pamphlets and booklets by Dr Henry Gilbert, The Biochemic Centre, Grantham, Lincs.)

Psionic medicine

This is based upon diagnosis of the sick person's blood-spot by Radiesthesia (medical dowsing). It is an infallible method of diagnosis (and consequently of treatment), but is a comparatively new 'therapy', and practised by only a few doctors in this country. For further information about it, see *Psionic Medicine* by J. H. Reyner, BSC, George Laurence, MRCS, LRCP, FRCS (Edinburgh) and Carl Upton, LDS. The book is published by Routledge and Kegan Paul.

For further information about Radiesthesia, see my book *Natural Remedies for Common Ailments*, published by C. W. Daniel Co.

CHAPTER TWENTY

Change Is Not
Necessarily Progress

Since the Second World War, people – and things – have changed a good deal, and, in my opinion, the change has not been for the better; indeed, it seems to me that a deterioration has taken place – in things, in people, in world health, in manners, and in morals. The standard of public service and of public entertainment has also deteriorated.

Take houses, for example – and food. The quality of both houses and food compares very unfavourably with that of forty years ago, and even more unfavourably with pre-1914–18 standard. Things, nowadays, are not made to last, as they were in those days and in the days of our parents and grand-parents. In those days, things of good quality and of attractive appearance were produced and sold at comparatively reasonable prices; nowadays, things are made of poorer materials and sold at ridiculously high prices. This applies not only to houses but to clothes and to most other manufactured articles, especially food-products, in all of which 'quality' is sacrificed to 'appearance', and, in the case of food, a longer shelf-life. Good, whole foods are turned into half-foods by 'processing' and by being tampered with by food-manufacturers, whose sole concern is to make big profits; they are *not* concerned with providing health-giving foods. These are the poeple – the food-manufacturers and food-technologists – who are chiefly responsible for the ill-health of the nation, though the food-growers, and the farmers who produce food-animals, are also partly responsible, for nowadays they, too, are prompted by the profit motive.

This (the profit motive) is at the back of all present-day forms of production, including food-production. The intensive rearing of food-animals (factory-farming), and the intensive growing of food-crops, has taken the place of old time-honoured methods of farming and of agriculture. Present-day methods of soil-fertilisation produce crops deficient in essential minerals, trace-elements, and vitamins. It follows, therefore, that the people (and the animals) that eat the crops will also be deficient in these essential substances, and that, as a consequence, their health will be adversely affected.

Present-day methods of farming (factory-farming) are highly unnatural and therefore detrimental to the quality of the flesh-foods produced (by the food-animals) on such farms. The poor quality of the animals' fodder, which, as explained above, is grown in improperly-fertilised soil, also contributes to the poor quality of the flesh provided by these food-animals.

Thus, it is obvious that a sick soil can produce only sick crops, and that sick crops can produce only sick animals and sick people. It is equally obvious that Soil Science (the study of the soil's construction and requirements) is therefore the basis of 'preventive medicine', i.e. the basis of good health and the prevention of disease in crops, in animals, and in humans.

For if the deficiencies in the soil are made good, this will make good the deficiencies in the crops grown therein, and thus in the animals and the human eaters of the crops. Unfortunately, present-day methods of fertilising the soil with artificial fertilisers do not make-good soil deficiencies; indeed, artificial fertilisers, if not used in conjunction with organic fertilisers, do more harm than good – they upset the chemical balance of the soil, and, although the result is an increase in the *quantity* and weight of crops produced, such crops are 'deficiency' crops, lacking in *quality*, i.e. in vital and essential minerals, vitamins, and trace-elements. (For further reading on this most important subject, see Lady Howard's book *The Earth's Green Carpet*; *The Living Soil* by Lady Eve Balfour, and books by Sir Albert Howard.)

If people eat 'deficiency' foods, they are bound, sooner or

F

later, to become ill, or at any rate to enjoy only sub-health, because deficiency foods do not supply the body-cells with what is essential to them for their maintenance, and so the cells deteriorate and die, or become diseased. Hence, the importance of eating properly-constituted foods, i.e. foods grown in properly-fertilised soil, and foods that have not been 'processed' or had the essential minerals, vitamins, and other vital substances removed. Such a food as white sugar is Public Enemy No. 1, and white flour is Public Enemy No. 2, because these foods have had their vital parts removed.

As for the deterioration in people's moral and spiritual health, this can perhaps be attributed, to some extent, to the deterioration that has taken place in their physical health due to 'deficiency' foods, mind and body being very closely inter-related and inter-dependent. Character is closely connected with, and can be radically influenced by, the type and quality of the food we eat. For example, the eating of flesh foods tends to make people hard, belligerent, and aggressive, lacking the 'milk of human kindness', lacking compassion for, and sensitivity to, all living things. A slight lack of magnesium in the blood can cause (and often does cause) mental instability, mental derangement, and even insanity.

Dozens of examples could be given of nutrient substances (or the lack of them) that cause mental and moral disturbances. White sugar, and all products containing it, is an outstanding example of a substance that causes havoc in the body, and, therefore, in the mind. If more than a very small quantity of it is eaten, it causes the sugar-content of the blood to drop to a dangerously low level (the condition is known as hypoglycaemia). Such a condition causes depression, fatigue, loss of interest in life, irritability, insomnia, a lowered resistance to disease-germs, and even, sometimes, suicidal tendencies.

Sugar in its natural state is dark brown; when it is refined, it is bleached with chemicals to make it white, and it is also robbed of its B vitamins. But, without these, it cannot be properly digested, so it has to leach the B vitamins out of the liver (and other organs of the body), thus creating a shortage of B vitamins in these organs, including a shortage of vitamin B12. This shortage of B vitamins, plus the low content of sugar in the blood, gives rise to the above symptoms. As soon as the intake of sugar is stopped (or even drastically reduced) the symptoms disappear. The explanation is as follows: when too much sugar is eaten, the immediate result is a sudden rise in the sugar-content of the blood; this rise causes an over-activity of the pancreas which produces an over-abundance of insulin, and this (the insulin) removes not only the *surplus* sugar from the blood but *all* of it, leaving the sugar-content of the blood very low.

There is a very close connection between sugar consumption and crime. Juvenile delinquents, who consume too much sugar, are often found to be suffering from low blood-sugar; so, too, are criminals.

Another reason for the deterioration in people's mental and physical health is closely connected with the hazards of meat-eating, for meat nowadays is often unhealthy, and, if not unhealthy, is full of harmful substances such as hormones, vaccines, antibiotics, etc, not to mention the animals' waste-products, which were on their way out of its system when it was slaughtered. Also, food-animals, in ranging over a wide area for food, tend to pick up poisonous plant-insecticides and radio-active fall-out, all of which are passed on to the consumer. Is it any wonder that our hospitals are full to overflowing? Every week, there are hundreds of cases of food-poisoning due to eating infected flesh-foods. Loss of working-hours due to such poisoning is twice as great as loss of working-hours due to strikes. Bacteriologists at St Bart's Hospital in London blame butcher's meat for an outbreak in 1970 of a new bacterial menace. Their study, entitled *Animal Sources of Common Serotypes of E.coli. in the Food of Hospital Patients*, which was reported in the *Lancet*, reveals their complete agreement about this. They report that E.coli. from such sources (from butcher's meat and from chickens contaminated with E.coli. from the bowels of the slaughtered animals) can colonise human bowels and cause serious intestinal and urinary troubles.

F I

Surely it is better 'to play safe' and eat only vegetarian foods. The world would be a healthier and a happier place (not least for the animals) if everyone did so.

As for doctors, nowadays, they are not doctors in the true sense of the word (the word doctor means adviser) they are merely 'disease-treaters'. In China, doctors are paid (by the State) only so long as they keep their patients in good health; when a patient becomes ill or diseased, the doctor treating that patient receives no payment until the patient is cured. This is as it should be. But in this country (and others in the Western world) doctors are not taught how to help their patients to *prevent* disease; they are trained only to *treat* disease when it has taken a hold on the body. The only form of 'preventive' medicine practised by them is vaccination (and other forms of immunisation), the hazards of which are considerable. (These hazards are discussed by Sir Graham Wilson, MD in his book *The Hazards of Immunisation.*)

A great many present-day orthodox doctors take no personal interest in their patients; they scarely listen to what the patient has to say, their whole attention being focused on form-filling; fellow-feeling for the patient is usually almost entirely lacking. Such doctors are therefore the very antithesis of what a real healer should be – of what Jesus Christ, the great healer, was. Real healers feel for, and *with*, their patients. This power to feel for others enables them to heal; it is an invisible power, but a very real one, and more powerful than any form of physical treatment, though of course physical treatment (in the form of corrected diet) should be given as well. The late Dr Edward Bach possessed this power. He healed with it, combined with his 'flower' remedies (remedies he made from plants which he found had healing powers over the mind). These remedies he gave to sick people whose emotions and mental processes were adversely affecting their physical health. (See '*The Bach Flower Remedies*' in my book *Natural Remedies for Common Ailments*, published by C. W. Daniel, who also publish seven books on and about the Bach Flower Remedies.)

CHAPTER TWENTY-ONE

Ancient Greek Philosophy and Medicine

Pythagoras (circa 500 BC) wore no clothing taken from animals; and he deplored the use of animals for food. He had strong convictions as to the importance of, and the necessity for, a harmless diet. He believed that men could be educated through their diet. He argued that, if they could be persuaded to be harmless and compassionate in their feeding habits, this attitude would eventually affect and permeate their lives and outlook, and their wars would consequently cease. Although a great scientist and astronomer, he considered that materialistic science was greatly inferior to the Divine Wisdom that enabled men to live rightly.

His strong feeling of 'a community of nature' with the lower animals caused him to plead eloquently with mankind to adopt a non-carnivorous diet, which he believed was natural to Man. He begged his fellow-men not to defile themselves by eating flesh-foods, seeing that Nature has provided mankind with banquets that involve no bloodshed – innocent foods such as grapes, grain, apples, herbs and vegetables, milk and honey – and he reminded them that only ferocious beasts such as tigers, lions, bears, and wolves demand slaughtered food. He expatiated on the enormity of sacrificing harmless animals to the gods; of tearing lungs, liver, or entrails from a living beast for the purpose of prognosis, and of such medical practices as cellular-therapy and animal experiments.

All such practices filled him with foreboding as well as horror.

He could see the retribution that must inevitably follow such practices, since every living creature is inextricably inter-related.

If his realisation of the kinship of all life, the eternal oneness of all things, was a more sentimental one than that of Darwin and his followers, it nevertheless led to that all-important reverence for life, the lack of which is now threatening the existence of humanity. He also foresaw that Man's scientific knowledge might outstrip his spiritual development, and that the application of such knowledge might lead to disaster (as I am convinced it *will*, unless there is a spiritual revival).

In his book *The Republic*, translated by A. D. Lindsay, MA (published by Dent), *Plato*, Greek philosopher, makes his friend *Socrates* his mouthpiece. In it, Socrates also points out that a vegetarian diet is essential if peace is to be enjoyed and war avoided. When describing the manner of life that should be lived by the citizens of the Republic, he says 'For food they will make meal from their barley, and flour from their wheat, and, kneading and baking them, they will heap their noble scones and loaves on fresh leaves, and drink wine after their repast, and sing hymns to the gods. Thus they will live with one another in happiness, guarding against the danger and poverty of war. They will have salt and olives and cheese . . . boiled dishes with onions and other vegetables, with a dessert of figs. And they will roast myrtle berries and acorns at the fire . . .'

He goes on to point out that land extensive enough to support people with simple vegetarian tastes will not be enough for pasturing herds of slaughter-food (cattle), and that it will have to be enlarged by acquiring someone else's territory, and to do that means warfare. Socrates does not pursue the subject of war, but it comes, he tells us, from the greed and covetousness and lusts of mankind, when men are not satisfied with simple living.

In his views on health, he not only forecasts the theory of psychosomatic healing in his contention that, for a real cure, the whole man must be treated and not just the affected part, but he also hints at methods of spiritual healing that were afterwards such a feature of the New Testament.

He speaks of Thracian physicians who cure by speaking to their patients 'words of the right sort' that heal the soul, on the assumption that, once the soul is healed, the lesser part (the body) must follow suit. 'This is the reason', he says, 'why most maladies evade the physicians of Greece – they neglect the *whole* – for, if the whole is out of order, it is impossible for the *part* to be in order. For all that is good and evil in the body and in man altogether is sprung from the soul. Therefore it should be the soul that is treated first and foremost if all is to be well with the rest of the body. And the treatment of the soul is by certain charms, and these charms are words of the right sort; by the use of such words temperance is engendered in our souls, and, as soon as it is engendered and present, we may easily secure health to the rest of the body or to one of its unhealthy parts.'

According to Plato (through Socrates), Virtue (the health of the soul) and physical health are inseparable, and, since he thinks the simple life and harmless vegetarian diet eaten by Pythagoras more virtuous than luxury and flesh eating, they must, he says, lead to better health. (What I think he means is that Virtue (health of soul) brings to its possessor a contented mind; a mind untroubled by pricks of conscience such as are suffered by people who know subconsciously that it is wrong to kill and eat flesh foods, and that, without a contented mind, what we eat and drink, however good it may be, will fail to bring us good health.)

He says that thought and emotion produce diseases that can therefore only be cured, or prevented, by the control and harmonising of thought. 'When the soul (mind) engages in battles of words carried on with controversy and contention, either in private or in public, it makes the body inflamed and shakes it to pieces, inducing cataarh.'

He advocated dieting rather than drugging as the remedy for physical ills. He said 'whenever anyone aggravates the disease by drugging, diseases many and grave instead of few and slight are wont to occur'. In other words, he recommended non-violence even in medicine, advice that might well be heeded by our modern advocates of wonder-drugs and antibiotics, who are continually perplexed by their side-effects that are often more fatal than the disease they were supposed to cure.

What he considered essential was spiritual healing. 'Ought not the doctor', he said, 'who is giving counsel to a sick man who is (or has been) indulging in a mode of life that is bad for health, to try first to get his patient to change his mode of life, and proceed with the rest of his advice only if the patient is willing to do this.'

Christ and Socrates both taught that Man must not stop short with obedience to authority, but must have the courage of his own convictions and act accordingly. Their ideas were in direct opposition to the religious beliefs of their own nation and form of government, and consequently both of them were condemned to die, and both died for the Truth. Socrates was tried, and ordered by the authorities in Athens to drink poison (hemlock) for corrupting the youth of the city by his philosophical teachings. (See *Lectures on the Philosophy of Religion* by G. W. F. Hegel, translated by Speirs and Sanderson.) The sublimity of Socrates in his martyrdom remains among the spiritual triumphs of the human race, as does the manner of dying of Jesus Christ.

Reverting to what Socrates said about first treating the soul of a sick man, it seems to me that soul *and* body should be treated, the latter via correct feeding. Maybe, in Socrates' day, the soil in which food was grown was more fertile and less exhausted than it is now, and, as a consequence, everyone ate better food, uncontaminated and unprocessed, and did not have to worry about whether or not he was getting adequate nourishment for his body. So that, in those days, perhaps ill-health *was* more likely to be due to sickness of soul than to deficiency foods (the present cause of so much ill-health). Nowadays it is due to soul-sickness *and* to soil-sickness, and the cure for both kinds of sickness can be learned from studying the right books. The *right* books will teach you self-knowledge, self-reverence, and self-control – the three qualities you need, Lord Tennyson said, to bring life to sovereign power. Indeed, there is nothing you cannot learn from reading, providing the wish to learn is in you. The trouble is to find the best instruction books. Yet this is not such a trouble as at first it may appear to be; the Head Librarian at any public library will be pleased to advise and help you, and will get suitable books for you, when he knows what you want to teach yourself.

First of all, you would be wise to teach yourself 'soil-health', so that you can grow your own food in soil that contains all the essential ingredients for health. This means knowing a bit about soil-science – the construction of soil, the making of compost, etc. For studying this, one of the best books is *The Living Soil* by Eve Balfour. Others are: *An Agricultural Testament* and *Farming and Gardening for Health or Disease* by Sir Albert Howard, *Gardening with Compost* by F. C. King, and *Commonsense Compost-Making* by May Bruce.

CHAPTER TWENTY-TWO

18th and 19th Century Philosophy

'There was a time when all knowledge was knowledge of God', *Hegel* the philosopher (1770–1831) says. 'Our own time, on the contrary, has the distinction of knowing all about everything, but nothing at all about God. Yet God is the one true Reality, the only Reality . . . God is everywhere present, and the presence of God is just the element of Truth that is in everything.'

In *The Basis of Morality*, *Schopenhauer* (1788–1860) says 'Boundless compassion for all living beings is the surest and most certain guarantee of pure moral conduct. The fact that Christian morality takes no thought for Beasts is a defect in the system.' Schopenhauer recognises that it is the Western departure from the concept of 'the unity' of all life that has led to this lack of compassion for other sentient creatures . . . It is the Realisation of the oneness and the unity of life, he points out, that produces Compassion, that is the actual explanation of Compassion, for it is the recognition of ourselves in all, and who does not love himself? Hence the admonition to love our neighbour as ourselves. How otherwise, Schopenhauer asks, can we account for the giving of even the smallest offering to those in need, with no other object than to relieve their affliction? But he is very dubious as to the possibility of arousing compassion in those who apparently do not possess it.

He identifies woman with compassionate love, saying that although she lacks justice, conscientiousness, etc, she surpasses man in loving kindness, and is more susceptible to compassion than men. 'Justice is more the masculine virtue, loving-kindess more the feminine virtue', he says. Both are necessary, the one tempering the other. 'But Compassion without Wisdom can be as dangerous as Knowledge without Compassion'. (Put in another way, this means, I think, 'Discretion is the better part of Valour'.) 'For in seeking to aid others, we often harm them for lack of the true wisdom that alone can reveal their true needs.'

But Schopenhauer's rejection of Vegetarianism – the obvious 'first step', as Tolstoy called it, on the path of a compassionate way of life – somewhat invalidates his sincerity as a philosopher and a humanitarian. But it does not invalidate the truth of all he said as to the necessity of recognising the unity of life, and the consequent duty of Man towards the lesser creatures. He himself was well aware of the oneness of all life, and he evidently learnt of the Wisdom-religion chiefly from Indian sources, because he tells how all old Indian dramas ended with the words 'May all living things be delivered from pain'.

CHAPTER TWENTY-THREE

Hydropathy

As used in ancient Greek and Roman Times

Hydropathy, the treatment of disease by water, was the foundation of all healing in Greek and Roman times. The Roman baths at Bath, built by the Romans during their occupation of Britain, are still there and still being used, although the great aquaducts that conveyed rain-water to the baths have gone. Hydropathy does not achieve much nowadays because the water being used is not rain-water with its high sun and oxygen content and its innate powers of cleansing and of healing. Its achievements are negligible (at any rate, in Great Britian) because it is not also accompanied by fasting (or semi-fasting) and diet-reform. At the Bircher-Benner Clinic near Zurich (and other such places on the Continent) it *is* accompanied by fasting and diet-reform, and is therefore more effective.

Hippocrates, the first real physician, who lived in Greece, 2,400 years ago, was of the opinion that all diseases are caused by a lack of oxygen in the blood and body-tissues. Oxygen, he said, is 'Lord of all' – essential not only for human life and health but also for animals and plant life, and even fire cannot live (i.e. burn) without it. He strongly advocated the use of rain-water, which he called 'sun-water', both internally and externally, together with the raw juices of fruits and vegetables. These, he said, by virtue of their oxygen and sun-water content, would give the body the necessary power (vitality) to cast out its own disease, which it would do, he said, through the excretory organs, especially through the skin by means of boils or abcesses. These occur only if disease *is* present in the body, and they should be helped to come to a head and discharge their toxins by the application of warm rain-water compresses, and by daily bathing in warm sea-water or rain-water. The treatment should be accompanied by much rest, fresh air, and sunlight, and an adequate but very light diet consisting mainly of fresh raw fruits, vegetables and vegetable juices, and, if thirsty, sips of rainwater. (The digestion of food takes energy; therefore, because energy is needed for self-restorative purposes, the sufferer should not eat to repletion.)

Rain-water is full of the electro-dynamic energy of the sun, whose power draws it up from the earth into the clouds, from whence it descends as rain. Fruits, vegetables, and plants are nourished by the rainwater in the soil in which they are growing, so they, too, are full of sun-water.

Rain-water contains not only solar energy, and 30 per cent more oxygen than tap-water, but also twice as much nitrogen, and nitrogen is essential for building and repair of body-tissues. Rain-water is lighter, purer, and less dense than tap-water, to which many chemicals are added, so it has the power to push and to penetrate into the minutest and remotest body-tissues and to supply them with oxygen, which is as vital to them as the food, vitamins, and minerals they receive. Indeed, it is thought by some eminent authorities that one of the causes of cancer could be a lack of oxygen in the bloodstream and in the tissues of the affected part.

The profound effect that rain-water has upon the human body is clearly, simply, and convincingly discussed and explained in a wonderful book called *Healing by Water* by T. Hartley-Hennessy, published by Essence of Health Publishing Company, whose address is PO Box 2821, Durban, South Africa (obtainable in England from C. W. Daniel Co Ltd). As the author says, one often hears the remark 'So-and-so has frequent boils and must therefore be in a very run-down state of health'. Nothing could be further from the truth. Anyone who has sufficient vitality to cast out poisons from his body by means of boils must be in excellent health. Sick people who have insufficient vitality to produce such outlets for toxins are to be pitied, for, if they *had* such outlets, they would soon recover their health. Such vitality is a power quite different from (and beyond) the healing ability of the medical man. It can be obtained only from Nature, from fresh air rich in oxygen, from oxygenated sun-water (as found in fresh fruits and vegetables), from rain-water, and from natural whole foods.

Faith and Hope and 'the Will to Live' are also powerful factors in the body's resistance to disease and its ability to summon up enough vitality to throw off disease. No doctor can help a man who has no desire to live, and the most skilled surgeon can only *set* a broken bone; it is Nature and one's own vitality that knits the broken ends together and heals the tissues.

Ancient and modern medicine are in direct opposition to one another. Ancient science taught that all healing would come from the sunlight (solar energy) contained in live plants and fruits, and in rain-water, combined with the innate recuperative powers of the body. Modern science teaches that healing can be effected by the use of man-made drugs. But these are foreign to the body (i.e. substances that do not enter into the composition of any of the cells) and simply give it *more* work to do, because they have to be ejected as rapidly as possible. They, therefore, hinder rather than help healing. Modern science also teaches that it is of no importance how dense water is, or how devoid of sunlight, oxygen, electrical forces and voltages from lightning, etc, nor how polluted it is, so long as it is made safe and drinkable by being chlorinated. In addition, water is being used in some parts of the country as a vehicle for sodium-fluoride (a substance that is supposed to harden children's teeth and to delay dental decay, but which has been proved to be harmful to many people). The practice of adding sodium-fluoride to water is tantamount to medicating it, moreover, it is enforced medication, since everyone is obliged to drink it in those particular parts of the country – and such a practice is unethical, and contrary to democratic principles.

From the moment that this sunless 'doctored' water is replaced by sun-rich rain-water, deterioration of body-tissues ceases and restoration begins. Bone repair, for example, is a very slow process; bones grow at the same rate as plants, and it may be many months before complete healing takes place. This applies not only to bones but also to other tissues and organs of the body. So, healing is slow, but sure.

In ancient times, hydropathy was used extensively by the Greek doctor Hippocrates, and other doctors, who placed dressings soaked in rain-water over any diseased part of their patient's body, in the hope of producing a boil or small eruption through which the disease might be drained from the body. However, there are people of such low vitality that even sun-water (used externally *and* internally) will not draw out the disease; in which case, something containing more sunlight than sun-water must be used, and that something is fruit-juice. The heat and drawing-power of an over-ripe fermenting apple (pulped) is miraculous; it will flatten varicose veins in about a week, and will draw the poisons from a diseased bone or tissue in a few weeks, if persistently used. All that is needed is a piece of clean linen, moistened with rain-water, on one half of which some over-ripe fermenting apple-pulp is spread, covered with the other half of the linen, and applied as a poultice to the affected area. It should be large enough to cover the area, and can be warm, very warm, or cold, the temperature does not matter, so long as it is exactly the temperature most comfortable to the patient. It must be changed several times a day, for the part must never be allowed to get dry. In ancient times, before the human race lost its self-cleansing and self-restorative powers, an inflamed appendix would in all probability have terminated as a large abscess on the surface of the abdomen, as a result of treating it in this way. Today, having forsaken natural living and a natural diet, people have lost the vitality to cast out their own poisons – such vitality is obtained only by observing Nature's laws and by living on natural foods and sun-water. It will give a man strength either to cast out his own disease, or, if surgery has to be resorted to, to make a rapid and complete recovery. For the greatest miracle of surgery is useless if the patient does not possess sufficient vitality to recover from it. Thus, one often hears the remark 'The operation was successful, but the patient died'.

CHAPTER TWENTY-FOUR

The Philosophy
of Longevity

'Man does not die; he kills himself' – so said Jean Finot, author of *La Philosophie de la Longévité*. What he said is true. Not only does Man get old and hasten his death by eating and drinking substances, such as cooked foods (especially flesh-foods), over-refined processed foods (all of which are 'dead' foods incapable of putting 'life' into him), but by allowing negative thoughts and emotions to take possession of his being. Youth is not a time of life; it is a mental condition, a precious state of mind. The age of the body is irrelevant so long as the mind, the emotions, and the instincts remain young. So not only must Man live abstemiously on the right (natural) foods; he must also practice mental hygiene if he wants to stay young. He must dismiss negative emotions (anger, worry, fear, etc) because any kind of psychological disturbance lowers resistance to disease. For, though we do not *die* of fear, or grief, or worry, they affect our system, undermining its powers of resistance. As Xavier Pelletier said: 'The depressing effects of physical conditions, of climate, and of daily intercourse with our fellow-men, must be combated by an unshakeable optimism. This is achieved by cultivating the will – a 'reasoned' will, which becomes an instinctive reflex act. We must master life, and dispassionately control our actions. This is the way in which we can ease our sorrows, suppress anger, eliminate from hatred all but the element of indignation that drives us to action, and know the joy of forgetting and forgiving.'

'Thou shalt not kill', we read in the Bible – and 'He who kills, kills himself' it says in the *Vedas*. Certainly this is true of the killing of animals for food, because eaters of flesh-foods are slowly killed by poisons and parasites that flesh-foods contain. Man was never intended to eat dead animals, which have to be cooked to make them palatable. The cooking does not destroy the poisons and parasites in them, but *does* destroy the digestive enzymes in their flesh, without which it cannot be *completely* digested or assimilated by Man. This means that the semi-digested portions set up putrefaction (a going-rotten process) in his large intestine, liberating toxic gases which poison his blood-stream and contaminate the nutritive juices that the blood is carrying round to all the organs and tissues of the body.

It is thought that, up until the Flood (about which we read in the Bible) Man's natural foods were the fruits of the Earth, but that, as a result of the Flood, which marked the beginning of the last glacial period on earth, he had to hunt and kill for food because vegetation on the earth was destroyed by ice, and was very scarce. This was the beginning of his downfall (healthwise). From this time forward, he also began to lose his natural instincts and his close contact with natural and cosmic forces. As a result, his life-span began to grow shorter, particularly as a result of switching from a vegetarian diet to a flesh-eating one. (See *Cosmos, Man, and Society* by Dr Szekely). The Patriarchs mentioned in the Bible, who lived before the Flood, lived to a great age – some to the age of 250 years, some longer.

Health is a vital equilibrium between external cosmic radiations and internal cellular vibrations. When this equilibrium is disturbed by any external (or internal) cause, a pathological state of the organism results, (a state of disease). In other words, it is only when our body-cells vibrate in harmony with natural radiations that we enjoy true health of body and of mind. Natural foods (the fruits of the earth) contain and emit natural radiations; they are classified according to the *kind* of radiations they contain and emit. For example, foods that grow under the ground (i.e. potatoes, carrots, and other root vegetables, also ground-nuts) have a predominance of terrestrial radiations.

Foods that grow on the surface of the earth (i.e. green, leafy vegetables) have a predominance of solar radiations. Foods that grow on trees (i.e. fruit, nuts, etc) have a predominance of cosmic radiations. Moreover, the character and value of these radiations is influenced and modified by seasonal radiations (i.e. by specific radiations that differ with the different seasons of the year). There are also foods that contain and emit not only terrestrial, solar, and cosmic radiations but other radiations; for example, milk, eggs, and honey contain animal radiations. The cell-vibrations of the animal from which the product comes can be transmitted to the product, and can be favourable or unfavourable to humans, who eat the product. An animal's cell-vibrations differ from the cell-vibrations of a human being, and these vibrations, which are unfavourable, are transmitted to a human-being when he (or she) eats animal flesh. And not only are unfavourable vibrations transmitted – animal flesh contains several poisons, in addition to waste-products which were on their way out of the animal's system when it was slaughtered, and all these harmful substances are transmitted to the consumer of animal flesh.

Animal flesh – also white of egg – contains Albumen (a nitrogenous compound, essential to life) but cooking makes it valueless, and not only valueless; it renders it harmful by decomposing it into toxic compounds, including uric acid. The best and most easily assimilated kind of albumen for humans is found in plants (vegetables), fresh fruits, nuts, cereals, legumes (peas, beans, and lentils), in seeds (sunflower, sesame, etc). Cow's milk is also rich in albumen, but nowadays milk is doctored with hormones and other harmful substances (it is also killed by pasteurisation), and therefore is not recommended as suitable food for humans. Moreover, its production involves such cruelty to the animals that give it, and to their off-spring. The calves are taken away from their mother (who obviously mourns their loss) immediately they are born. They are fed on artificial milk-products, never tasting a drop of their mother's milk, in highly unnatural conditions, on factory-farms, and the bull-calves are slaughtered at twelve weeks old. Cheese is, of course, made of milk, and its production involves additional cruelty, in that a substance called rennet is needed for making it. Rennet is obtainable only from the stomach of a calf, which therefore has to be killed to obtain it. (Cheese made without animal rennet is, however, obtainable from health-food shops. It is made by Marigold Foods Ltd.)

CHAPTER TWENTY-FIVE

Cosmos, Man, and Society

by Dr E. Szekely

Summarised Parts of his 'Thoughts on Transmigration'

When life has ceased, the ordinary forces of the inorganic world are no longer the servants of the organic framework, as they were during life; they become its masters. Oxygen, the scavenger of the living body, becomes the sovereign lord of the corpse. Atom by atom, the complex molecules of the tissues are broken into pieces and reduced to simpler and more oxidised substances, until the soft parts have evaporated (chiefly in the form of carbonic acid, ammonia, and water) leaving only the bones and teeth. But even these dense tissues are unable to offer permanent resistance to water and air. Sooner or later, the organic base, which keeps the earthy salts united, decomposes and dissolves; the solid tissues become friable and are reduced to dust. They finally dissolve and are spread over the waters of the earth, just as the gaseous products of decomposition disperse in the atmosphere.

These transformations cannot be followed with any certainty; they are more various and more extensive than those imagined by the sages of antiquity who believed in transmigration. However, it is probable that sooner or later some of the atoms, if not all, scattered in space, will reassemble in new forms of existence. The action of the rays of the sun upon the vegetable world introduces the wandering molecules of carbonic acid, water, ammonia, and salt into the composition of plants. The plants are eaten by animals; animals eat one another; man eats both plants and animals. So it is quite possible that the atoms which at a given moment formed part of the troubled brain of Julius Caesar may today have entered the brain of an Alabama negro or a farmyard watch-dog.

Thoughts on Nutrition

We must start with a fast of two or three days, or, in the case of illness, with one of a week or fortnight, during which the inferior elements which have accumulated in the organism over a period of many years will be set in motion and eliminated, mostly through the urine [in the form of sediment].

The regeneration of the system and the renewal of all the cells is achieved by the dissolvent and eliminative effect of the organic salts of fruit and vegetables. This regeneration is feasible, even at the age of 80 or 90. It is only unfeasible in the case of old people who have shrunk a lot.

Our blood forms the source of energy for our regeneration.

Elimination of inferior elements is quickened by exercise in the open air, by conscious breathing exercises, and by sun and water baths. Fasting is more bearable if, after two days, we continue with a little fruit, and especially if we take some intestinal douches at the start.

If we get rid of the products of the kitchen (i.e. cooked foods) we very quickly end our illnesses. If we masticate thoroughly and eat raw foods, we cannot exceed the natural limits in quantity, because the natural elements in them fix the amount of them needed by the organism. The less we need of a food, the more perfect that food is. That is why wheat and fruits are the most perfect forms of food. Three ounces of wheat, soaked in water for 24 hours, if well masticated, are sufficient for an organism. Artificial foods always deceive us and make us eat more than we ought, because our organs and senses cannot function normally when fed on these unnatural products. We can never establish the precise amount of these foods because they do not form the preconditions of our existence. Even the smallest amount leads us to old age and death, a small amount less quickly than a large amount.

Meat is exclusively the diet of the lower carnivorous animals. For humans it is more dangerous than nicotine, because nicotine is a single poison; meat contains *eight dangerous* poisons. In countries such as Great Britain, where meat is the staple article of diet, only one person in every 100,000 lives to the age of 107. Of every 100,000 new-born children, 30,000 die in the first year of life, 11,000 in the second year. This high rate of infant mortality is caused by the complete intoxication of the mother's organism by the poisons in meat, by her inferior liquids poisoning the child while it is in embryo. The stronger ones hold out longer in the struggle against toxins, but their number is diminishing, and it is only the most abstemious who manage to attain to a more advanced age.

There are a large number of centenarians in Bulgaria, due, it is thought, to the fact that the majority of the population eat no meat. The basis of their frugal diet is plain (i.e. unpasteurised sour milk, milk-products, and vegetables). Those who live entirely on cereals (chiefly brown rice) and milk products are even more abstemious in their use of milk than are the rest of the people. (They are called Macrobiotes, and most of them live to a great age, usually over 140.)

Cooked foods are incapable of insuring or maintaining the vitality of our organism. A *cooked* vegetarian diet (even an abstemious one) can prolong life by only very little. Neither bread, cooked vegetables, nor milk products can prevent the slow and progressive degeneration of our cells, old age, and death. The most important precondition of longevity is a fruitarian diet and periodical fasts. A fast of as little as 36 or 48 hours once a week or once a fortnight, is enough, on the basis of a natural diet, to make us immune to every disease. The special capacity of the blood for elimination of toxins increases with each fast. For instance, if we fast for two days completely (or with fruit only), we shall find in our urine, after some hours, a deposit of sediment. This waste-material (which causes illness and old age) is dissolved and eliminated by our blood which the fast has vitalised. The more we fast, the greater the success of our efforts to regenerate ourselves. During the first two or three weeks of a long fast, the urine is copious and contains much sediment, but gradually both decrease, and finally the sediment disappears altogether. If we live for a time on fruit after a fast of this kind, we can be sure of real improvement. Death and gravitation will have lost their influence in our organism. Fruit, being the noblest food, provides the source of energy for the improvement, leading to that degree of perfection when Man will be able to assimilate the elements of Nature (i.e. to live on air). However, it is a mistake to think that large amounts of fruit (or of any other natural food) give more strength and vitality. An excessive quantity of *any* food not only overloads the organism with unnecessary work but the surplus is dissolved in the blood and changes into fermentative and decaying matter, which, even with a perfect diet, leads to inferior function. Our organs and senses undergo progressive improvement upon a *frugal* fruitarian diet, and function properly. If we fast on one (or two) days a week on a fruit diet and also obey the other laws of Nature, we can approximate to the longevity of the Patriarchs of the Bible. It is recorded that Adam lived to be 950 years old; the shortest lived of them was Enoch who lived to be 365 years old. It is thought that they owed their longevity to living on a completely natural diet of the fruits of the earth; to their constant contact with natural elements and cosmic radiations; to their harmonious social and moral life; also to the fact that they lived *before* the Flood, after which Man was obliged to hunt for his food and to eat animal flesh instead of a vegetarian diet, owing to a destruction of vegetation, of fruit trees, and of forests, by a great glacial extension. Starting from this time, Man began to lose both his natural instincts and his close contact with natural and cosmic forces, and the average length of his life began to grow shorter.

As already stated, the most important precondition for

maintaining and improving our vitality is the fast. One other practice which contributes to the revitalisation of our organism is internal douching (bowel wash-outs).

The effect of having lived on an unnatural diet for many years is that our intestines are full of putrid matter and inferior fermentations. In such an environment, a large number of parasites and worms, visible *and* invisible, multiply. In most cases, evacuation of the bowels is not regular or normal, and the waste-matter is never entirely discharged from the intestines, and so inferior stratified layers are formed on the walls of our large instestine.

Nutritive juices are absorbed into the organism through the inner surface of these walls, and consequently they reach the blood tainted with this fermented material that adheres to the walls. As a result, all our nutritive juices are infected, and this condition increases our liability to disease.

On a cooked diet (even a vegetarian one) it may be several months (even years) before our vital energy can rid the body of all the fermented contents and parasites of our large intestine. This is because they are able to continue to live on the contents of the intestine derived from vegetarian food, and so they can form the permanent precondition of all contagious diseases. That is why internal wash-outs must be used for several days at the beginning of our new régime, at the same time keeping to a diet of fruit only. After the putrid matter, fermentations, hardened faeces, and parasites have been eliminated, our intestinal system will regain its vitality and elasticity, particularly if, at the same time, we adopt a natural vegetarian diet and start the renewal of our soul. Normal absorption of nutritive juices is then a certainty. We must continue the daily bowel wash-outs for a whole month if our new way of life follows long years of an unnatural, flesh-eating, cooked-food diet. Even later on, when we are leading a natural life on natural foods, it is a very sound plan to take a daily douche for a week, three or four times a year. It can be taken morning or evening, but not less than eight hours after a meal.

The gravitation of the earth has a most remarkable influence on all rotting matter. Corpses become the food of the earth. But the earth's gravitation also attracts all the inferior products stored in *living* organisms; so do water, air, and sun simultaneously. Of all the elements in Nature, earth has the greatest dissolvent power. The dissolvent power of water and of air is increased by the action of the sun.

Disease is always caused by putrefaction of matter in the organism, and substances in a state of putrefaction are most rapidly dissolved in the earth; so if we put sick people to lie on wet earth and cover all but their heads to a depth of 6 inches, the remarkable dissolvent force of the earth will make itself felt in half an hour. This treatment (it is called Geotherapy) is particularly effective in external cancers, wound fractures, infections of the blood, and infections caused by snake or dog bites. In these cases (bites) a large lump of wet earth must at once be put on the bite for a few minutes and the victim made to lie on the wet earth, covered completely with earth (except for his head), and here he must stay for some hours. All danger is thereby averted. Clay compresses can be used for cancerous sores, also for rheumatic thickenings; they should be applied every night for at least a month.

The electric forces of the vital elements are the source of perfect vitality. It is these that keep the vital fire alive and develop the electrical force of our body cells. Only by taking advantage of such electric forces can we achieve, in and through our organism, perfection. On the other hand, if we impair the vitality of our organism by absorbing unnatural foods which have been destroyed by cooking, we shall have introduced inferior processes into our system, and our vital juices will have been impaired and will have been dissipated through our sexual organs. Though we may abstain and may suppress sexuality, we do not get rid of the principal cause of it, which is perpetual violation of the laws of nutrition. For, if life is unable to work towards perfection in the body, it must always leave that body to try to achieve perfection by the creation of a new individual. This tendency appears from generation to generation until the objective is gained by the creation of a perfect descendant.

Individuals working towards perfection must never degrade love into a pleasure. They must devote it to the great purpose of evolution, by the creation of superior generations. Concentration of mental forces and a natural life will enable the will to triumph over sexuality. The new individual created by the concentration of superior thoughts will inherit not only the capacities of his generators but also superior energies. Those who begin the new life on the basis of only superficial knowledge, without understanding the totality of natural law will never get complete results; they cannot expect to be cured by only one (or more) of the forces of Nature. Real seekers after Truth seek to improve themselves by progressively acquiring the capacity for optimal orientation based upon an *all-round* knowledge of natural law.

'In our new life, sleep assumes a new significance, as it is simply a process of detoxication. As the poisons in our system gradually grow less under a new way of life, our need for sleep will also diminish, but the amount of sleep we need must be guided by the promptings of our organism. During deep sleep, our eliminatory organs are most active, and the circulation of the blood is undisturbed by any outside or conscious influence; accordingly, it eliminates all the products of oxidation through the appropriate channels. The instinctive and unconscious activity of our sub-conscious nervous system *Is* the Law, because our conscious (cerebro-spinal) system (the violator of the Law) is asleep. The more natural our life, the less sleep we need.

The final objective of the higher man is the attainment of perfect vitality, i.e. the ability to assimilate the elements of Nature (insolated air and water) in order to achieve perpetuation of his regeneration. Man re-creates and improves himself by means of transformations based on knowledge of the Laws of Nature.'

Professor Woodruff of Yale University has proved by experiments on monocellular organisms that *cells are immortal* if kept under the right conditions. He kept them in a nutritive liquid, and this liquid he renewed from time to time because, not only did it become deficient in nutrition as the organisms consumed the nutrition, but it became saturated with the waste-products and the products of oxidation proceeding from them. These waste-products, unless removed from time to time, are consumed by the organisms; they poison them, and they die. But if the nutritive liquid is periodically renewed, the organisms proliferate, mutliplying by division, and continue to live for a period that corresponds to a quarter of a million years of human life. His experiment proved that if monocellular organisms are immortal under favourable conditions, then the higher organisms (humans), made up of millions of cells, ought also to be immortal. According to Carrel, a surgeon of the Rockefeller Institute, the cells of the human organism *are* everlasting. Their mechanism is such that they are capable of eternal life, unless prevented by external circumstances. This is true, our cells are eternal like those of monocellular organisms, but, on account of their position in the organism, they cannot completely eliminate the unavoidable by-products of the vital processes, and these become poisons to them. The monocellular organisms, living in their nutritive liquid which is periodically changed and cleaned, can clean out their poisons completely and are consequently immortal under such favourable conditions. The cells of Man are continually being poisoned; the many different diseases to which Man succumbs are the result. In the final analysis therefore, the cause of death in Man is always poisoning of the cells of which his body is composed.

According to Crile, a Professor at Cleveland University, living cells always contain electricity which gives them the necessary force for vital activity. The cells are little electric batteries. While they are young, they have plenty of electricity, and they eliminate the toxic waste-products of their food easily and rapidly. Later on, poisons accumulate in them which lessen their electricity and their capacity for eliminating these poisons. If the cell loses its electricity altogether, it dies.

All these scientists recognise that the cells which constitute our bodies are immortal. At the same time, they declare that our bodies (the aggregate of these cells) *must* die, because the by-products of life which poison them cannot be completely eliminated, that it is the gradual accumulation of poisons and the progressive loss of electricity which inevitably lead our aggregate of cells (i.e. our body) to old age and death.

CHAPTER TWENTY-SIX

The Ageing Process

As Dr Heinz Woltereck says in his book *A New Life in Old Age*, living and developing are one and the same thing; so, since people now live longer than they lived a few hundred years ago, they have more chance of reaching spiritual maturity, and thus of ensuring a good eternity. As one grows older, there is a lessening of the vital interests, due to a decrease in the physical urges, and this sets free other forces – intellectual and spiritual forces – that can develop and can produce a comparatively new and valuable phase of life; particularly so in the field of mental energy.

In *Life Begins at Forty* by W. B. Pitkin (a book now out of print) the thesis is developed that we only become our true selves in later life; that until we reach the second half of life, when certain physical processes have run their course and when we are consequently able to achieve the mental and spiritual detachment that leads to Wisdom, we are not able to become our true selves. Certain it is that 'sex' is a yoke round the neck of many people, and that, as soon as they reach an age when they are no longer saddled with it, they begin to develop spiritually and mentally. This does not apply of course to everyone – many people develop spiritually and mentally during their youthful years while at the same time enjoying physical pleasures – but, for those to whom it does apply, the problem of how to increase the life-span, so that they have more time on Earth in which to develop spiritually, is an important one.

In *How To Prolong Life* by Dr Charles de Lacey Evans, we

read how to do this. The author (who wrote the book in 1879) advises living on a diet composed entirely of raw fruits and nuts, these foods being Man's natural foods, the foods he ate in pre-historic days, the days before the first Ice-Age when, because the Earth was covered with ice, he had to take to hunting and killing for food. The author says that of all the foods available to Man, fruits are the least 'clogging' and there-fore the least harmful to the human system, because it is clogging of the system that shortens the life-span. Fruits con-tain much smaller amounts of 'earthy compounds' (clogging substances) than any other food, and it is these earthy com-pounds (chiefly phosphate and carbonate of lime) that clog the system, diminishing the calibre of the larger arterial vessels and eventually obliterating the small vessels (the capillaries), thus hastening the ageing process.

To retard the ageing process we should therefore avoid foods which contain a high content of 'earthy compounds' (such as cereals and things made from cereals) and live entirely on fruits and nuts, which contain only a very low content. 'Earthy-compounds' are derived from the soil in which the cereals, etc, are grown; they are taken up by the plant, becoming part of it, and becoming part of us when we eat the plant. They accumu-late in our system, and, together with the waste-products of body-metabolism, cause the ossifications of old age, and even 'natural' death.

Next best to fruit and nuts for increasing the life-span is fish, and, next to fish, dairy produce; then vegetables (especially green leafy ones); then peas, beans, and lentils; last of all cereals. (Dr Evans was evidently not a vegetarian – we vege-tarians do not approve of eating fish or any dead creatures.)

The author of the book also says that it is of vital importance to drink only distilled (or natural spring) water, and that foods should be eaten *raw* as far as possible, because cooking devita-lises them and changes them chemically, making them less able to be properly assimilated by the body (which seems to me a very good reason for not eating flesh-foods, which *have* to be cooked to make them palatable).

CHAPTER TWENTY-SEVEN

Credo

I believe that if the desire to achieve something, or to be something, is long enough and strong enough, you will either get what you desire, or good reason why you have not got it will sooner or later be revealed to you and will enable you to be content without it. God works in a mysterious way.

I believe that my own small personal life is bound up with the life of every living, breathing creature in the universe, and that I cannot hurt any living creature without harming myself; that cruelty is a sort of boomerang which, when you throw it, comes back and hits you.

I believe that Man has no right to exploit animals as he does. They are dumb, defenceless creatures, entirely at his mercy – part of God's wonderful creation – and Man should treat them mercifully. Christ said 'Thou shalt not kill'. I believe that He meant this to apply to *all* living creatures.

I believe that there is no such thing as necessary cruelty, any more than there is necessary sin; that vivisection, often practised with the greatest cruelty, in the hope of securing some possible (though doubtful) benefits to humanity, can never be justified or bring good in its train. Man fears death above everything else, and feels that *anything* is justified – even unspeakable cruelty – if there is the remotest chance that it may postpone his day of death. The animals on which he experiments, (testing life-prolonging drugs, etc) are helpless, but their Creator rules the universe, and will, I believe, punish Man for his cruelty to them.

I believe that nothing that is perfectly natural is ever really vulgar; that it is only pretence and artificiality that are vulgar.

I believe that the way to get things is to give, not actively to give, but to do so passively, by not struggling and snatching. Like a wave when you are not looking, happiness creeps up to take you by surprise.

I believe that to study things of the mind and intellect is to look merely into the mind of Man, but that to study 'matter' is to look into the mind of God, the Creator of all matter.

I believe that strength of character requires not only strong emotions but a strong control over them, and that a sense of proportion and a sense of humour are necessary for preventing one's emotions from becoming tinged with sentimentality.

I believe that none of the many emotions which Man is capable of feeling is wrong in itself; it is wrong only if uncontrolled.

I believe that, in order to achieve a working contentment, either our senses or our soul should be temperate in desire; there must be compromise in the satisfaction of the demands of each.

I believe that, in conformity with the Law of Attraction, which rules that 'like attracts like', every sincere seeker after Truth will be instinctively drawn towards the things and the people that will help him to find what he is seeking. 'Seek and ye shall find' is advice based upon this natural law.

I believe that there is nothing you cannot achieve if you tune-in to the divine wave-length. Only by means of meditation and prayer, coupled with a deep desire to find it, will you ever find this wave-length, but, once found, it will be a never-ending source of inspiration and help to you.

I believe that peace is the old-age pension of the soul; that it is earned by contributing generously and unselfishly towards a fund of things that give pleasure and help to other people; that thus to contribute is the main purpose of living.

I believe that the power of thought is the greatest power in the world; for good or ill. So –

'Let your secret thoughts be fair;
They play a vital part and share
In shaping words and moulding fate:
God's system is so intricate.'

Books for Further Reading

An Agricultural Testament, Sir Albert Howard, Oxford University Press

The Earth's Green Carpet, Lady Howard, Oxford University Press

Fertility Farming, H. Newman Turner, Faber & Faber

Food is Your Best Remedy, Dr H. Bieler, Faber & Faber

The Master Key to Health, Rasmus Alsaker, Harrap

Soil, Grass and Cancer, Andre Voisin, Crosby Lockwood

Nature's Medicine, Richard Lucas, Neville Spearman

Nature Hits Back, McPherson Lawrie, World's Work

Natural Remedies for Common Ailments, Constance Mellor, C. W. Daniel Co

Our Synthetic Environment, Lewis Herber, Jonathan Cape

Our Poisoned Earth & Sky, J. I. Rodale, Rodale Press

The Blood Poisoners, Lionel Dole, Health for All

The Handbook of the Bach Flower Remedies, Philip Chancellor, C. W. Daniel Co

The Stress of Life, Hans Selye, Longmans

Inside Yourself, Louise Morgan, Hutchinson

Food Reform Cook Book, Vivienne Quick, Health for All

Kingston Nature Cure Clinic Recipes & Methods, C. Leslie Thomson, C. W. Daniel Co

Animal Machines, Ruth Harrison, Vincent Stuart

Silent Spring, Rachel Carson, Penguin Books

Crimes Against Creation, Marie Dreyfus, The author

In Pity and In Anger, John Vyvyan, Michael Joseph

Books for Further Reading

These We Have not Loved, V. A. Holmes Gore, C. W. Daniel Co

On Behalf of the Creatures, J. Todd Ferrier, Vegetarian Society

Why Kill for Food?, Geoffrey Rudd, Vegetarian Society

The Perfect Way in Diet, Anna Kingsford, Vegetarian Society

Vegetarian Cuisine, Isabel James, Vegetarian Society

Ethics of Diet, Howard Williams, Richard James

Gospel of Peace of Jesus Christ, Edmond Szekely, C. W. Daniel Co

The Gospel of the Essenes, Edmond Szekely, C. W. Daniel Co

Philosophy of Compassion, Esme Wynne Tyson, Centaur Press

The Civilised Alternative, Jon Wynne Tyson, Centaur Press

Food for a Future, Jon Wynne Tyson, Centaur Press

Food Fit for Humans, Frank Avray Wilson, C. W. Daniel Co

Food for the Golden Age, Frank Avray Wilson, C. W. Daniel Co

Handbook of Health, Constance Mellor, Mayflower Books